T0296750

TELESTROKE

TELESTROKE

LATISHA KATIE SHARMA
Associate Professor
Neurology
University of California, Los Angeles
Los Angeles
CA, United States

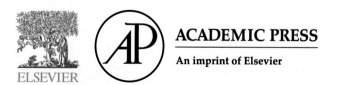

ELSEVIER

ACADEMIC PRESS
An imprint of Elsevier

Academic Press is an imprint of Elsevier
125 London Wall, London EC2Y 5AS, United Kingdom
525 B Street, Suite 1650, San Diego, CA 92101, United States
50 Hampshire Street, 5th Floor, Cambridge, MA 02139, United States
The Boulevard, Langford Lane, Kidlington, Oxford OX5 1GB, United Kingdom

Copyright © 2021 Elsevier Inc. All rights reserved.

No part of this publication may be reproduced or transmitted in any form or by any
means, electronic or mechanical, including photocopying, recording, or any
information storage and retrieval system, without permission in writing from the
publisher. Details on how to seek permission, further information about the
Publisher's permissions policies and our arrangements with organizations such as the
Copyright Clearance Center and the Copyright Licensing Agency, can be found at our
website: www.elsevier.com/permissions.

This book and the individual contributions contained in it are protected under
copyright by the Publisher (other than as may be noted herein).

Notices
Knowledge and best practice in this field are constantly changing. As new research
and experience broaden our understanding, changes in research methods, professional
practices, or medical treatment may become necessary.

Practitioners and researchers must always rely on their own experience and knowledge
in evaluating and using any information, methods, compounds, or experiments
described herein. In using such information or methods they should be mindful of
their own safety and the safety of others, including parties for whom they have a
professional responsibility.

To the fullest extent of the law, neither the Publisher nor the authors, contributors, or
editors, assume any liability for any injury and/or damage to persons or property as a
matter of products liability, negligence or otherwise, or from any use or operation of
any methods, products, instructions, or ideas contained in the material herein.

Library of Congress Cataloging-in-Publication Data
A catalog record for this book is available from the Library of Congress

British Library Cataloguing-in-Publication Data
A catalogue record for this book is available from the British Library

ISBN: 978-0-12-824161-5

For information on all Academic Press publications visit our website at
https://www.elsevier.com/books-and-journals

Publisher: Nikki Levy
Acquisitions Editor: Melanie Tucker
Editorial Project Manager: Tracy I. Tufaga
Project Manager: Kiruthika Govindaraju
Cover Designer: Alan Studholme

Typeset by TNQ Technologies

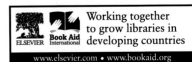

Working together
to grow libraries in
developing countries

www.elsevier.com • www.bookaid.org

Contents

List of figures

List of tables

CHAPTER 1

History of telestroke

Telemedicine also referred to as "telehealth" or "e-health" is defined as use of telecommunication and information technology to provide clinical healthcare from a distance. However, there are several definitions which are not well integrated and are often used interchangeably. Telehealth encompasses a broader array of digital healthcare services. To understand the nuances, it is essential to define the terms. The definition of the term telemedicine as outlined by the World Health Organization is, "The delivery of health care services, where distance is a critical factor, by all health care professionals using information and communication technologies for the exchange of valid information for diagnosis, treatment and prevention of disease and injuries, research and evaluation, and for the continuing education of health care providers, all in the interests of advancing the health of individuals and their communities" [1]. The Health Resources and Services Administration (HRSA) of the US Department of Health and Human Services defines telehealth as "the use of electronic information and telecommunications technologies to support and promote long-distance clinical health care, patient and professional health-related education, public health and health administration. Technologies include videoconferencing, the internet, store-and-forward imaging, streaming media, and terrestrial and wireless communications." In an effort to simplify the definitions, telemedicine can be defined as the practice of medicine remotely (patients are geographically separated from the clinician) and telehealth is a term that encompasses all components and activities of healthcare and the healthcare system that are conducted through telecommunications technology.

Telemedicine likely began its path in ancient Greece where early attempts to establish rudimentary communication with smoke signals and light reflections established connectivity between patient and physician [2]. In their book, *History of Telemedicine*, Rashid Bashshur and Gary Shannon discuss the theme of connectivity and traced the transformation and evolution of telemedicine over the decades [2–4]. From drums to pigeon signals, human civilization has been able to communicate and convey information over long distances. In the 19th century, Alexander Graham

TeleStroke
ISBN 978-0-12-824161-5
https://doi.org/10.1016/B978-0-12-824161-5.00001-3

© 2021 Elsevier Inc.
All rights reserved.

1

Bell patented the telephone, a device for electronic speech transmission. Long-distance telephone links began appearing in the 1880s and several technical innovations since that time have led to creating the platform for the advancement of telemedicine as it exists today. An article published in 1879 in the *Lancet* described the transmission of medical knowledge over the telephone and conducting doctor's appointments through the telephone in order reduce the burden of in-person visits [5]. In 1906, William Einthoven, inventor of the electrocardiogram, published a paper on the telecardiogram where impulses would be transmitted through telephone wire from the patients in a hospital some distance away [6]. The US military telegraph network communication was used during the Civil War for ordering medical supplies as well as communicating deaths and injuries on the battlefield. In the 1920s, the radio was used to give medical advice to clinics on ships. A Radio News Magazine from 1924 features an illustration of a doctor attending to a patient via video call, under the headline "The Radio Doctor—Maybe!" [7] (Fig. 1.1). According to one review, the first reference to telemedicine in the medical literature appeared in 1950 [8]. The article described the transmission of radiologic images by telephone between West Chester and Philadelphia, Pennsylvania and subsequent creation of a Canadian teleradiology system in the 1950s [9—12]. In the 1960s, the University of Nebraska used a two-way interactive television to transmit neurological examinations, group therapy consultations, speech therapy, diagnosis of difficult psychiatric cases, and education and training

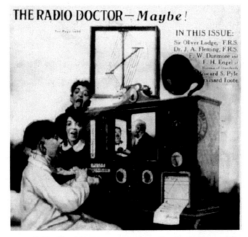

Figure 1.1 The cover of Radio News magazine, April, 1924 with an illustration of a doctor attending to patient via video call.

[13–16]. The National Aeronautics and Space Administration (NASA) played a crucial role in advancing telemedicine as it began to send astronauts into space. Physiologic monitoring with continuous transmission of reactions of the cardiovascular were transferred by one-way telemetry downlink in Mercury and Gemini space programs [5]. In collaboration with the US Indian Health Service, NASA worked on the Space Technology Applied to Rural Papago Advanced Health Care (STARPAHC) project to provide telemedicine access to an American Indian reservation via telecommunication links similar to the one used for space stations [17].

Despite the advances in technology, the high costs of maintaining a program and programs failing to become financially independent and profitable led to decreased interest and few telemedicine programs persisted [18–21]. Toward the end of the 1980s, technical progress and cost-effective strategies led to a regrowth of telemedicine programs and renewed interest in telemedicine applications for patient care [22,23]. Our connected world communicates by telephone, text messages, and email. Often these communication methods are used to notify patients about their test results or discuss medications with their physician and we call 9-1-1 to report medical and other emergencies. Interestingly, most people do not consider this a form of telemedicine. The Telecommunications Bill of 1996 contained measures with relevance to telemedicine directed specifically at assuring universal communications services at affordable rates for rural, high-cost, or low-income areas, including instruction relating to such services, to any public or nonprofit healthcare provider that serves persons who reside in rural areas at rates comparable to those charged in urban areas. Congressional interest in telemedicine is reflected in Senate/House Ad Hoc Steering Committee on which cosponsored a 1994 conference to develop a consensus agenda for telemedicine and health informatics [4]. During the 103rd Congress, at least 22 pieces of legislation specifically related to telemedicine were introduced [24].

Today, information technology and telemedicine plays a central role in advancing healthcare [24]. Electronic medical records and patient portals allow medical information to be disseminated efficiently for medical providers and patients. New medical applications (teleradiology, telepsychiatry, telestroke) and technologies such as digitized and compressed data improved bandwidth information transfer, better industry standards, and advanced telemedicine units have driven the growth of telemedicine [19]. Telemedicine has grown rapidly and has become a path to virtual integrated care of specialty departments, hospitals, private doctor offices, home healthcare, and the patient's home. Currently, over 76% of US hospitals connect with patients and consulting practitioners at a distance through the use of video and other technology [5]. Several states have been awarded grants by the Department of Health and Human Services for several different rural pilot telemedicine projects. However, there are several key factors that continue to limit the use of telemedicine: high costs, current lack of reimbursement by insurers, lack of clinical standards, scheduling difficulties, and time limitations. A review of prospective controlled clinical trials involving distant medical technology (including telephone contacts and consults) concluded that electronic communication with patients enables greater continuity of care by improving access between physicians and patients, in areas of preventive care, and in the monitoring of several chronic conditions such as diabetes and hypertension [25].

Telemedicine has shown great promise in changing the trajectory of acute stroke management. It supports decisions at hospitals without stroke care expertise to improve patient access to recommended treatments. Levine and Gorman introduced the term telestroke in their editorial published in *Stroke* in 1999 [26]. Telemedicine for stroke, "Telestroke," uses state-of-the-art video telecommunications to facilitate remote cerebrovascular specialty consults. Telestroke is considered one of the most successful applications of telemedicine, bringing the experience of stroke experts to hospitals lacking appropriate stroke expertise. Telestroke was initially pioneered in Boston where remote neurologic assessment was demonstrated to be reliable and increased the rates of thrombolysis [27−31]. Telestroke has grown significantly in the past 2 decades and its role in the management of acute stroke patients has changed care worldwide. Telestroke enables patients to be remotely evaluated, allowing optimal treatment and management even in clinically underserved areas and removing geographical disparities in access to specialty expert care (Fig. 1.2). The majority of vascular neurologists and emergency physicians surveyed agreed that telestroke reduces geographical differences in stroke management and is superior to telephone consultation [32].

In the United States, approximately 800,000 people experience a stroke each year. Stroke is the fifth leading cause of death and a leading cause of serious long-term disability. Stroke reduces mobility in more than half of stroke survivors aged 65 and over [33]. It is one of our nation's most expensive diseases to treat, estimated at $41 billion per year [34,35]. In order to decrease the burden associated with stroke related to long-term disability (lowered ability to perform daily tasks, the cost of care, and lost productivity), we need to improve a patient's clinical outcome by rapid assessment

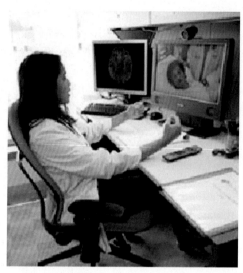

Figure 1.2 Acute telestroke consultation. Telestroke physician provides an acute telestroke consultation to an emergency physician at a local hospital where a patient with an acute stroke syndrome presented. She is able to conduct a video-enhanced neurological examination as well as view the patient's computed tomography (CT) scan.

and treatment. In the United States, there are $\approx$ 4 neurologists per 100,000 people, although many parts of the United States lack access to acute stroke services entirely [36–39]. The emergence of the neurohospitalist (a neurologist whose primary professional focus is hospital-based medicine) was expected to mitigate the problems of emergency department and inpatient stroke coverage. However, continuous 24 h emergency coverage remains difficult for many remote, rural, and underserved urban emergency departments and hospitals [40,41].

One treatment option for acute ischemic stroke is systemic thrombolysis treatment, using tissue plasminogen activator (tPA). Thrombolysis treatment dissolves the clot that is obstructing blood flow to the brain, preventing permanent damage and is therefore associated with favorable outcomes. There is a narrow treatment window for thrombolysis treatment; it must be delivered within 3 h of symptom onset, and it requires specific neurological expertise in order to guide the decision-making regarding ideal candidates for the treatment. The only Food and Drug Administration—approved treatment for acute ischemic stroke, intravenous recombinant tissue-type plasminogen activator (rt-PA), should be administered within 3 h of the onset of stroke symptoms. Recent guidelines recommend that selected patients can be treated up to 4.5 h after symptom onset [42–44]. Treatment of ischemic stroke with rtPA reduces neurological impairment and disability, hospital length of stay, and percentage of patients going to rehabilitation and nursing homes [45]. Patients who receive tPA within 90 min of symptom onset are almost three times as likely to have favorable outcomes 3 months after a stroke than those who do not receive tPA [46]. The American Heart Association estimates that only 3%–5% of ischemic stroke patients are treated with thrombolysis [47]. In a review of Medicare billing records of 4750 hospitals and almost 500,000 cases of AIS over a 2-year period, 64% of surveyed hospitals never administered tPA. Patients were less likely to be treated with tPA in the Midwest and southeast [48]. One-third of Americans live more than an hour from a primary stroke center and only about 27% of stroke patients arrive at the hospital within 3.5 h of symptom onset [47,49]. There are currently only four neurologists per 100,000 persons in the United States, and even emergency departments in urban and suburban areas are not able to have stroke neurologists readily available [50].

There are several reasons for the low rates of administration of tissue plasminogen activator; however, a major barrier has been timely access to stroke experts. These experts are typically located at major centers and patients in rural or remote areas are unlikely to receive thrombolysis treatment unless remote physicians are able to obtain rapid expert help in order to guide decision-making and treatment planning. Many emergency physicians are hesitant to accept the sole responsibility for administering intravenous thrombolysis for acute ischemic stroke and may not utilize acute stroke treatments such as tPA [51,52]. Nearly 90% of rural emergency departments would be receptive to joining a telestroke network and treating patients with acute stroke with thrombolysis if a vascular neurologist could provide a telemedicine consultation [53,54].

Telestroke systems enable thrombolytic treatment to be administered in community and rural hospitals, and facilitate the appropriate transfer of patients with complex conditions (who require critical care services such as neurosurgical or intraarterial interventions) to a comprehensive stroke center. Clinical trials demonstrating that endovascular thrombectomy can substantially improve outcomes for patients with large vessel occlusions further expanded the acute ischemic stroke treatment window. Identifying patients likely to benefit from a higher level of care at more specialized centers and initiating an immediate transfer are critical functions of a telestroke network [55]. tPA treatment is usually initiated on site using telestroke and patients are then transported to a primary stroke center or CSC [27]. Compared with patients directly admitted to the stroke center, outcomes of patients with remote supervision of intravenous tPA initiation and subsequent transport to a regional stroke center are similar [56].

A study of four urban hospitals in Illinois found that their utilization of tPA increased by two to six times after telestroke was implemented [57]. Several studies demonstrated that adherence to intravenous thrombolysis protocols could be improved by implementing telestroke networks [58]. Thrombolysis rates were significantly greater after telemedicine implementation without an increase in the rate of incorrect treatment decisions [59]. Telestroke systems allow the clinician to reliably assess the National Institutes of Health Stroke Scale (NIHSS) and take a few minutes longer than an in-person evaluation [29,58,60]. The remote stroke evaluation was also reliable if performed by a telemedicine naïve examiner or a nurse practitioner (guided by a vascular neurologist) [61,62]. In a randomized study conducted in California, telestroke decision-making was superior to consultation by telephone with respect to administration of tPA to patients [58]. Correct treatment decisions were made significantly more often in the telemedicine group than in the telephone consultation group (98% versus 82%, OR 10.9, 95% CI 2.7−44.6). There was no difference between the groups in 90-day clinical outcomes, although this study was underpowered to detect differences in functional outcomes [58,62]. Taken together, these therapies provide important treatment options for clinicians, significant reduction in disability for patients, and reduced long-term costs for healthcare systems.

Telestroke networks have improved efficiency and resulted in more consistent standardized treatment within the narrow treatment time frame. The first telestroke network connected rural facilities in Swabia (TESS network) and Bavaria (TEMPiS network) to central hubs with extended stroke care capabilities [63−65]. These pilot studies demonstrated the feasibility of a large-scale telestroke network in facilitating remote use of thrombolysis [30,31]. In 2009, the American Heart Association/American Stroke Association published companion articles that specifically reviewed the evidence for telemedicine within the stroke systems of care and made recommendations for implementation [38,39]. The 2009 policy statement included guidelines that contained 14 recommendations, 9 of which were based on Class I evidence. They emphasized the value of telestroke to support the immediate assessment of stroke severity via the NIHSS and other instruments and its equivalence to that of a bedside assessment, the review of brain computed tomography (CT) scans by stroke specialists to decide about thrombolysis eligibility and urgent decisions about thrombolysis. Telestroke systems can also facilitate ongoing follow-up and consultation by remote stroke specialists during the patient's hospitalization and facilitate improvements across all aspects of patient care (increase use of thrombolytic therapy, endovascular therapy, inpatient management, rehabilitation, discuss reliability, validity, efficacy within each area). Current acute stroke guidelines continue to endorse the use of telestroke for these indications [55,66]. (see Figs. 1.3 and 1.4)

Key components to implementing an effective Stroke System of Care include the need to factor in the nature of the First Responders (e.g., fire/police/volunteer, BLS, ALS, Paramedic, Flight Nurse). This includes incorporating EMS assets effectively, taking into account EMS by ground and air, and mobile stroke units (MSUs). Utilizing regionalized point of entry routing plans for suspected stroke destination. A tiered accreditation or designation of stroke centers that includes the recommended levels of Basic, Acute Stroke Ready, Primary and Comprehensive centers. These

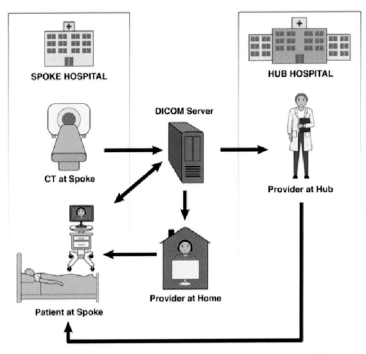

Figure 1.3 Organizational model of stroke telemedicine [67].

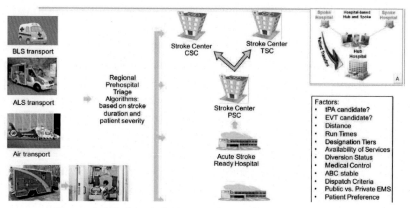

Figure 1.4 Prehospital triage pathways for acute stroke [68].

systems should encourage high levels of participation in National QI programs with recognition for performance to ensure that systems are based on infrastructure and performance.

Additional innovations include the use of telemedicine in MSUs to improve treatment with thrombolysis in the prehospital setting. Faster treatment with recombinant tissue-type plasminogen activator can be achieved by moving the diagnosis and drug delivery into the prehospital setting using a MSU, a specialized ambulance equipped with a CT scanner, point-of-care laboratory, and a team including a CT technician, paramedic, nurse, and physician, linking patients in the ambulance to the emergency department. In 2012, the first randomized trial results regarding treatment of stroke patients in an MSU versus hospital were published. This study demonstrated that acute ischemic stroke could be treated with tPA faster [69]. In 2015, a larger study in Berlin integrated the MSU with the fire department and was successful in treating large numbers of patients safely and quickly [70]. In 2021, Ebinger and colleagues provided the first convincing evidence that MSUs, compared with conventional ambulances transporting patients to an emergency department, treat more patients with acute ischemic stroke, treat them faster, and improve their outcomes [71].

Stroke education through the use of Internet-based initiatives for healthcare professionals and patients has also improved with the use of telestroke [26]. The education and supervision of residents and fellows can be enhanced with telemedicine. An attending physician's direct participation via telemedicine in the evaluation of a patient in the emergency department can improve the efficiency and timeliness of patient care. The capability to archive telemedicine sessions provides a library of simulation scenarios that can be reviewed in an educational setting to evaluate real-world patient encounters. Telemedicine applications can address several core training competencies such as patient care, communication, professionalism, and systems-based practice [72]. Telestroke could also improve the rate of recruitment and enrollment of underrepresented populations of patients into clinical trials of acute stroke treatment and can help with identification and follow-up of patients, allowing for a more diverse and representative sample of patients [73]. The use of telemedicine to obtain consent in the prehospital setting and emergency department setting is a promising solution to some common challenges to acute clinical trials [74].

Telestroke has since moved beyond the prehospital and emergency department setting and is widely used in the inpatient, rehabilitation, and outpatient settings. The integration of a virtual stroke unit provides ongoing follow-up and consultations by stroke specialists with a structured aftercare stroke system. Since 2001, stroke performance measure guidelines have been published and sponsored or cosponsored by the American Heart Association/American Stroke Association [75]. Implementation of quality improvement initiatives based on performance measure data has been associated with improved timeliness of intravenous tPA administration after acute ischemic stroke, reduced rates of in-hospital mortality, and an increase in the percentage of patients discharged home [75]. Systematic measurement of the quality of stroke care in the United States began in the early 2000s with the funding of the pilot Coverdell stroke registries and the establishment of the Get With The Guidelines—Stroke program, one of the largest ongoing clinical quality registries in the world [76]. A collaborative network for acute stroke care using ongoing data collection and review can lead to significant improvements in care and increase compliance with performance metrics. Both neurologists and emergency physicians agree that telestroke can reduce the geographic disparity in stroke treatment [32,77]. Development and initiation of telestroke-specific quality improvement measures can lead to refinement and expansion of telestroke networks in the prehospital and discharge settings [78].

In the United States, multiple hospitals have made commitments to their communities to improve access to stroke care by becoming part of local, regional, and multistate telestroke networks. Compared to no telestroke network, a telestroke system can result in more use of tPA and stroke therapies, more patients discharged home independently, and overall cost-savings for the network of hospitals [73,78—83]. Each network hospital has telestroke technology that links their emergency department physicians and nurses directly with a team of stroke experts available 24 h a day, 7 days a week. Several studies have demonstrated the applicability and feasibility of telestroke networks in acute stroke care [84—90]. The number and extent of telestroke networks continue to grow in the United States and throughout the world. Monitoring practice quality and outcomes becomes essential to maintaining a high level of performance and ensuring that patients receive the full potential benefit of this approach. This integrated approach is cost-effective from both societal and individual hospital perspectives. Moving forward, telestroke will serve as a foundation on which multicenter studies will be developed and facilitated in an ongoing effort to firmly establish the value of telestroke in healthcare. Telestroke is a powerful and innovative platform to enhance the care of stroke patients and brings a new horizon in modern day healthcare.

CHAPTER 2

Practical telestroke: setting up a practice

Teleneurology has led to a dynamic shift in neurologic care in the inpatient and outpatient setting, particularly in stroke. A telestroke practice usually incorporates the use of a combination of synchronous and asynchronous technology but may also include remote monitoring. Synchronous services (e.g., Zoom for Healthcare Skype for business, Updox, Doxy.me) allow patients and clinicians to interact in real time, allowing for clinical history taking and physical examination. Asynchronous (e.g., 98Point6, Conversa, Ro) refers to a "store and forward" process in which there is delayed communication. Clinical data (photos, videos, or data files) are digitally collected, electronically transmitted, and later reviewed by a clinician. Asynchronous technology is inexpensive and works well for triage but does not allow for a provider to take a history or conduct an examination [91—93]. Remote monitoring may be assessed with real-time evaluation of a patient's clinical status or by review of personal health data collected remotely [94]. (See Table 2.1).

Outpatient telestroke practice

Several key elements are required to implement and maintain a successful virtual neurovascular clinic. The practice must closely match the onsite experience and be able to provide consistent care for all patients. Patients receive benefits of time-saving and reduced travel expenses. A physician also saves time, gets exposed to a more diverse patient population, and has fewer missed appointments and cancellations. Prior to implementation, prerequisites include determination of interest and need, administrative and clinical support, credentialing/legal capabilities, technology, and sustainability. It is essential to clarify if a telemedicine clinic would fill a need in your area or specialty as upfront costs and time invested may not be sustainable if patients do not use the service. Current technology using web-based software which merges with the clinic's existing equipment (e.g., desktops, tablets) has lowered the startup costs. (see Fig. 2.1).

TeleStroke
ISBN 978-0-12-824161-5
https://doi.org/10.1016/B978-0-12-824161-5.00002-5

© 2021 Elsevier Inc.
All rights reserved.

Table 2.1 Types of telestroke setup and utilization details.

Type of model	Description	Effectiveness
Mobile chat or messaging apps	Mobile chat or messaging apps have been used to share clinical data and clinical care guidance Some applications may not be secure or compliant with HIPAA requirements, data may be vulnerable	• Allows the multidisciplinary care teams to be immediately notified of the arrival, location, and stage of evaluation for stroke patients. The communication on this application can be secured with end-to-end encryption. • in the outpatient setting allows for quick, safe discussions with healthcare provider, making or updates regarding appointments, better approachability
Audio/visual telestroke platforms	Two-way, interactive, real-time video sessions at a bandwidth sufficient to allow for synchronous patient care	• This model enables the neurologist to perform clinical history taking and physical examination, interact with patient and family as well as healthcare providers
Virtual reality, augmented reality, telepresence	An enhanced version of reality is created by the use of technology to overlay digital information on an image of something being viewed through a device Encounter can occur in an artificial environment which is experienced through multisensory stimuli	• Interactive real-time feedback in the ED or home/outpatient setting for acute stroke or telerehabilitation • Seamless hands-free wearable devices
Email consultation (e-consult)	The neurologist receives an email referral, and then decides whether advice alone was appropriate, or whether visit was indicated	• This was proven to improve clinical effectiveness, lower direct costs, and increase productivity

Table 2.1 Types of telestroke setup and utilization details.—cont'd

Type of model	Description	Effectiveness
Remote monitoring devices	Real-time evaluation of a patient's clinical status or by review of personal health data collected remotely	• Provides real-time data tracking and assessments, in which biometric data can be monitored at the patient's home and electronic health records
Store and forward	Delayed communication. Clinical data (photos, videos, or data files) are digitally collected, electronically transmitted, and later reviewed by a clinician	• Simple, reliable, inexpensive, and effective method of asynchronous communication

Adapted from Patel UK, et al. Multidisciplinary approach and outcomes of tele-neurology: a review. Cureus 2019;11(4): e4410.

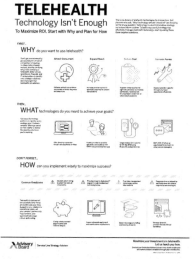

Figure 2.1 Outpatient telehealth practice setup.

Outpatient telestroke practices routinely use nonvideo technology, which can include telephone or secure messaging via mobile apps (e.g., WhatsApp, Skype, Backline, LunaHealth) to provide information or advice, transfer digital imaging or laboratory results, monitoring patient status, appointment setup and notifications to improve accessibility. Physicians, nurses, and other medical personnel speak with patients and families without the expense or inconvenience of an office visit for the patient or a home visit for the clinician. To reduce avoidable office visits, many health plans have established telephone advisory programs, staffed primarily by nurses, to provide patients with information, assessments, and recommendations for routine medical problems [58,82,87,93,97−101]. Some patients may not have access to telecommunication devices. To bridge the gap, telecommunication devices should be covered as medical necessity and allow for accessibility accommodations such as closed captioning (Fig. 2.2).

For more in-depth assessment, practices can use flat screen, high definition models, and three-dimensional images with assistive devices to help with the examination. Basic needs include a secure Internet connection, a video platform, and technology support. High-definition televisions, cameras, and robotic devices assist in more precise diagnosis by allowing closer examination of pupil size, facial features, and subtle deficits; however, these upgrades can lead to increased expenses. There are otoscopes, stethoscopes, and ophthalmoscopes that can connect to a mobile device such as the iPhone to assist with the evaluation. Some of these units are able to communicate with each other but other equipment may use proprietary communication technology. Several electronic health record (EHR)

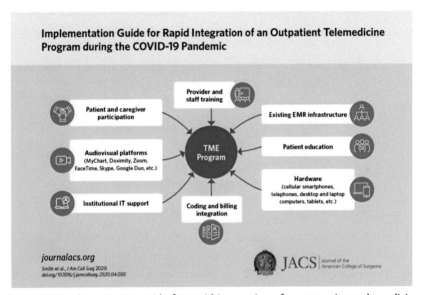

Figure 2.2 Implementation guide for rapid integration of an outpatient telemedicine program [96].

systems have integrated telemedicine into its platform allowing the healthcare provider to chart and document as they evaluate the patient while reducing cost.

There are limited communication standards regarding equipment but reliable broadband Internet service is a must, both for the provider and the patient. High speed options are more widely available and less expensive. The amount and speed of the Internet connection determines the video quality and speed of data transfer. A basic business broadband connection should be sufficient at about 50−100 Mbps (Megabits/second). A basic televideo can be found through third-party vendor where the patient will use a home computer or smart phone to communicate with the physician. More expensive solutions involve provider control of the interface on both ends. Qualified computer and technical support are necessary for the success of the program. The support can be virtual or in person depending on resources, but physician access at all times is critical. They need to be available to help with technical and hardware problems which may occur during a clinic day to prevent interruptions to patient care [102,103].

There are a variety of options for platform setup. These include the simpler "dual connect solution" where the physician speaks to patient on one monitor and document in the HER in another. This allows for the lowest cost and greatest ease of access for physicians. Partially integrated solutions allow for built in virtual visits and enhances the patient's experience with virtual waiting rooms, automatic preauthorization, and documentation for the physician directly into the EHR avoiding loss of data. The most expensive, fully integrated platform allows the patient video visit portal directly within the EHR. All documentation flows into the practice EHR [103].

Telemedicine interactions must comply with the Health Insurance Portability and Accountability Act (HIPAA) of 1996 and other regulatory requirements. Maintaining patient privacy is a critical element in providing care via telemedicine. General web-based software does not usually meet standard accepted measures for ensuring a secure and private transmission. Most telemedicine technologies create a point-to-point encryption between the devices or use virtual private network (VPN) tunnels for privacy of the connection. Most telemedicine software and videoconferencing companies (e.g., AMD Global Telemedicine On-Demand Visits, AmWell, BrightMD, MDLIVE, SOC Telemed, Teladoc Health, VitelNet, and Zipnosis) use encryption to ensure remote visits are protected. Healthcare providers should conduct the evaluation in a well-lit space where the interaction cannot be seen or overheard, maintain professional attire and conduct the evaluation in an environment that mirrors an in-person visit. Patients should be encouraged to be in a safe, secure, quiet space if possible [99].

Expedite and streamline the training process, create a basic how-to video for the clinical team. This training video can be created with an iPhone or professional videographer, depending on budget and overall use. Your video becomes a quick reference guide, and decision tree, for your team but should include how to use the selected technology, types of patient encounters to be performed, when to deploy the technology, how to alert coworkers that you are engaged in a telehealth encounter and how to be informed if there is a matter requiring urgent attention [94]. Adapt existing clinical protocols and incorporate components for referrals and scheduling, preconsult preparation, remote site coordinator duties, clinical sessions (including evaluation and treatment suggestions), and post-examination procedures. All telemedicine protocols should outline processes at distant and provider sites to ensure Health Insurance Portability and Accountability Act (HIPPA) compliant procedures and transmission of approved Notice of Privacy Practices, consents, and other required paperwork. A printed How-to Quick reference guide should be written in an easy to understand format and available in the office and as a pocket guide as well.

A designated telemedicine coordinator familiar with the telemedicine procedures (how the technology works, process expectations) and scheduler with appropriate administrative support is a key component of a telemedicine practice. It is important that they are well trained and equipped. A script or FAQ sheet about the service should be made available so that the scheduler is comfortable explaining the transition to a virtual visit to patients and have consistent and informative conversations with patients. A scheduler should work with the patient before, during, and after the telemedicine encounter. When a referral is received, the scheduler consults with the provider team and advises the patient concerning preferred medical history or records, and which tests (if any) need to be performed prior to the appointment. Next, the scheduler gathers information concerning the patient's current contact information so that intake paperwork can be delivered. At that time, a tentative date and time is set for the consultation, dependent on the completion of paperwork before the clinic date. Paperwork may include proper consent forms, history, and insurance information. After the paperwork is returned, the scheduler confirms the appointment time with the patient. After the consultation, the scheduler assists with scheduling any requested follow-up appointments. Connection should be tested for compatibility and back-up plans should be in place in case of technology failure. While telemedicine can reduce no-shows and cancellations, incorporating it into a practice workflow often requires rerouting of routine practice and retraining of staff. If there is a technology issue, use telephone triage to reduce patient frustration and help mitigate physician liability. (See Fig. 2.3).

Understanding the regulatory requirements, credentialing and legal aspects will lead to a seamless transition within a practice. These may vary based on institution, local, state, and federal level. Most states require licensure of providers in each state they plan to practice, including for telemedicine clinics. This requirement is particularly important if Medicaid or Medicare is to pay for the services. If the program partners with rural hospitals and clinics, extra credentialing may be required [99]. Many decisions will be cost and potential use driven, while others will be based on coding needs and documentation.

It is also important that the clinical team practice within limits they find comfortable and acceptable. All ethical standards and integrity of a practice must be upheld to ensure that patients get the best care possible [99]. Personal comfort with exam and communication will also factor into a positive experience with telemedicine visits. The visit is generally best

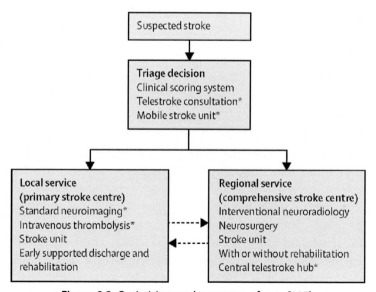

Figure 2.3 Optimizing stroke systems of care [115].

suited for very focused patient evaluation and does not require a detailed physical examination. Proper "webside" manner is important during a telestroke encounter. Clinicians must maintain a professional appearance and avoid wearing complex patterns which can cause a kaleidoscope on camera. Patients endorse comfort with professional workwear such as white lab coat or scrubs. It is important to maintain situational awareness and act as if the camera is always on even if encounter designated as audio only. Anecdotal experience during the pandemic describes many situations where a staff member set up an audio only encounter only to later realize that the camera was turned on or clinicians had their audio on but were unaware that patient was on the line and able to hear their private conversations.

Sustainability is a major challenge although telemedicine is becoming more mainstream and increasingly covered by insurance companies. Assessment of metrics can help gauge the strength of the program. These metrics can include volume of telemedicine encounters, track individuals or practice to understand what works or if retraining is needed, track the cancellation and no-show rates and diagnosis [94]. Marketing of the program to patients is also important to sustainability. Social media encourages a two-way conversation with news from your facility, and feedback from patients. Some practices use a paid search to help patients find a clinician, when they are not already connected to a clinical practice or hospital. Brochures and flyers can also inform patients and referral sources about a practice's telehealth services [91].

Emergency department and inpatient practice

Videoconferencing stroke services have developed for more than almost two decades, with the major impact of care in rural areas by increasing access to thrombolysis for stroke patients, and improving long-term functional outcomes. Real-time, audio–video tools connect a clinical encounter guided by a stroke expert to physicians and patients in the emergency room. The stroke expert can determine whether to administer thrombolytic therapy or if transfer to a stroke center is required. The telestroke consultant must also have real-time access to neuroimaging, in order to guide clinical decision making. Systematic review of telestroke programs has found reduced mortality, beneficial health outcomes, and treatment reliability through video consultations. It has been shown The National Institutes of Health (NIH) Stroke Scale can be reliably performed, that neurologists can reliably interpret unenhanced brain computed tomography (CT) images for stroke diagnosis, and that tPA can be safely administered through teleneurology [54,58,82,83,86,87,104,105]. Several studies have demonstrated the applicability and feasibility of telestroke networks in acute stroke care [87,89,90].

There may be a need to address resistant providers and perceived increased complexity of telestroke. Strengthening relationships with telestroke consultant and ED providers, standardizing the telestroke consult process, and expanding the goals and roles of the program are vital to program success [106]. The American Telemedicine Association delineated telestroke guidelines regarding the successful operation of a telestroke system [107]. As outlined in the guide, there should be agreed-upon key roles and responsibilities and support from key stakeholders (hospital administrators, IT, clinical personnel, human resources, legal, and finance). The telestroke hub (distant site) should have a physician medical director who acts as a champion for the program and supervise administrative issues at both hub/distant and spoke/originating sites. The director should be able to supervise the administrative issues that commonly arise. The director often has specialty training in stroke and should cultivate the program by developing and maintaining relationships with spoke/originating telestroke sites and designing evidence-based care pathways. A telestroke champion at the spoke/originating site should be designated and aware of the telestroke protocols, telemedicine technology platforms, criteria for transfer to a site providing higher levels of care, referral arrangements, cerebrovascular disease, and telemedicine in general.

A telestroke program manager is based at the hub/distant site, and interacts with the medical staff services, IT, and legal offices at both the stroke center and at all supported spoke/originating sites/hospitals. This manager should ensure contracts are in place, licensure and credentialing are current, training and education are being delivered, billing and coding are accurately performed, quality measures are in place, quality assurance processes are being followed, and overall administrative oversight is provided for the telestroke program, under the medical director's supervision. A successful program also requires an ED stroke champion. The ED physician roles at telestroke spoke/originating site facilities should include familiarity with telestroke alert criteria, processes and procedures for initiating a telestroke call and consultation, telemedicine technology platforms, and stroke clinical protocols. ED nurse roles should include interaction with emergency medical system (EMS) personnel, intake of an acute stroke patient, triage, recognition, rapid evaluation, and stroke treatment protocols. Qualifications for roles of other contributing telestroke providers should be focused on optimal acute stroke care, telemedicine technology proficiency, troubleshooting, and familiarity with working effectively within regional stroke systems of care [107].

Other hospital provider roles may depend on the scope of the practice, but could include hospitalists, neurointerventionalists, intensivists, and radiologists. EMS personnel, physician assistants (PAs), advanced practice nurses (nurse practitioners), laboratory and radiology personnel, IT administrators, or other personnel who are committed to training clinical providers and providing quality oversight to the program may also be part of the telestroke program. The originating and receiving facilities will need a designated 24/7 IT liaison with specialized training in the hardware, software, and clinical algorithms associated with telestroke services as this role is critical to the seamless functioning of the technology. Small or rural hospitals lacking the IT resources may need the distant site or the telemedicine technology vendor to provide support to the originating site. Oversight and metrics should include a review of consecutive telestroke cases for timeliness of emergency evaluations, correctness of clinical decision-making, appropriateness of treatment delivery, and comprehensiveness of post-ED care for the patients not transferred to the stroke center [107]. Some healthcare systems develop distributed networks where telestroke is available at multiple originating sites through arrangements with an independent corporation or an affiliated network of telestroke providers. Typically, there are transfer agreements for endovascular therapy or subsequent stroke care that are defined to facilitate evidenced-based stroke management.

Quality improvement

Donabedian first described the three interconnected constructs of structure, process, and outcomes and is credited with defining a useable organizational framework for measuring healthcare quality and outcomes in modern-day health systems [55,108]. According to Donabedian, structural measures denote the attributes of the settings in which care occurs. Structural measures describe the characteristics of the healthcare system itself, including system capacity (e.g., number of hospitals, bed size), human and physical resources (e.g., availability of specialists, staffing ratios, number of wards/units), and organization structure (e.g., hospital referral networks, stroke units, stroke teams) [108—110]. Process measures denote what is actually done in giving and receiving care. They describe the complicated processes and actions required to deliver care and are most often linked to specific recommendations from clinical guidelines [108,110]. Outcome measures denote the effects of care on the health status of patients and populations. Ideally, outcome measures should reflect those outcomes that are important to patients such as death, disability, functional status, and quality of life and should be measured in a time window that is relevant to the actual delivery of care [55,108,110].

Continuous quality improvement is a key element for any successful telestroke program. Systematic collection and analysis of quality data has been shown to improve the quality of stroke care. Quality measures help assess and quantify the overall function of telestroke systems. Many hub hospitals have stroke certification through standards set by the Joint Commission on the Accreditation of Healthcare Organizations process. Evaluating the capacity of the healthcare system, staffing ratios of specialists, availability of specialized units, and equipment for any telehealth network systems. It is important to identify process measures but these have not been clearly defined for telestroke. Identifying traditional stroke pathway elements such as door to needle times and door to consult time can help improve the telestroke pathway. Successful telestroke programs will also need to define and measure patient and or system-related outcomes. Identification of stroke mimics and morbidity and mortality data are important in telestroke-treated patients. As with traditional stroke programs, utilization of the 90-day modified Rankin scale (mRs) is recommended. Assessment of patient and provider-related outcomes and data collection regarding patient characteristics, NIHSS score pre/posttreatment and before discharge, length of hospital stay, discharge disposition (home vs. rehab vs. subacute rehab), readmission rate, and complications are also important to capture [107,111—113]. Feedback regarding technology including technical difficulties, failures, and limitations should be continuously monitored, documented, and analyzed promptly. Universal telestroke guidelines regarding definitions of times in the stroke chain-of-care, protocols for consultant notification, and standardization of telestroke network protocols are important considerations for sustainability of telestroke models [107,111—113]. There are several telestroke models that have been described. These include the following models listed below [107,111,112]. The hub and spoke with external sites and third-party distribution models are the most commonly used models within telestroke [107]. (See Tables 2.2 and 2.3).

Table 2.2 Telestroke models.

- Hub and spoke single healthcare system
- Hub and spoke with external transfer agreements
- Third-party distribution model: telestroke services are provided to multiple originating sites through arrangements with an independent corporation or an affiliated network of telestroke providers
- Horizontal hubless network: interconnected sites within a large hospital system where teleconsultations during off-hours are performed by local neurologists of all hospitals involved in the network in rotation
- Supervisory training model: academic teleneurology programs to assist trainees within the hospital system

Table 2.3 Potential telestroke quality metrics to measure and track performance.

Effectiveness	• Increase in thrombolysis rates • Accuracy of diagnosis and correct decision-making (preliminary and final discharge diagnosis)
Safety	• Rate (%) of symptomatic hemorrhage
Performance	• Median time to emergency department arrival • Median time to stroke team activation and response • Median time to imaging and imaging review • Median time to diagnosis and eligibility for acute treatment determined • Median time of patient arrival to initiation of IV thrombolysis • Median time of arrival and departure at originating site • Median time of arrival at receiving site • Median time of patient arrival to groin puncture
Technology	• Monitor failure of technology and impact on clinical decision-making
Imaging	• Image quality, transfer of images • Monitor equipment failure
Disposition	• Percent of patients requiring transfer from spoke to hub
Morbidity and mortality	• Outcomes similar to those treated at a stroke center
Satisfaction	• Patient satisfaction with consult • Remote provider satisfaction • Teleneurologist satisfaction

Telestroke consultation workflow

The typical workflow for a telestroke consultation begins with the patient arrival to the spoke site who has a suspected stroke. The remote site physician performs the initial assessment and activates the telestroke consult. Simultaneous laboratory and imaging orders are initiated. The teleneurologist evaluates and examines the patient, reviews the neuroimaging, and decides on treatment with thrombolytic therapy. The treating physician determines if transfer is needed for endovascular or neurosurgical intervention and initiates the transfer process. The teleneurologist would close the loop with the remote site physician and discuss the plan of care. The term "drip and ship" is often used to describe transfer from spoke to hub sites, where the thrombolytic therapy is started at the spoke and patient is emergently transferred for higher level of care [114]. (See Figs. 2.3 and 2.4).

There are different ways to configure delivery of telestroke based on the needs of a particular program. While this could be telephone based, evidence suggests telestroke is superior to telephone consultation alone [116]. Practice models include teleconsultation alone with advisory services and the referring hospital maintains responsibility and liability for the patient, tele thrombolysis where the remote neurologist decides on thrombolysis and is responsible to varying degrees for the patient's course, typically in the context of a preexisting agreement between hospitals or via an integrated telehealth system with exchange of patients, information, and therapeutic suggestions between centers involved in acute stroke care, often with disseminated responsibilities and no clearly dominant hub [30,38,39]. Many remote hospitals have stroke care capacity, but lack around the clock stroke coverage. In these circumstances, teleconsultations for mild to moderate strokes may result in "drip and keep," where tPA is administered and patients remain at the local hospital with local neurology coverage. Use of this virtual stroke unit allows the patient to be closer to home and family

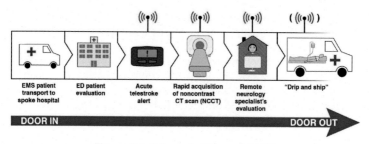

Figure 2.4 Drip and ship model [67].

support and reduces the burden of transfer costs for the patient and health system. Studies such as the Telemedicine in Stroke in Swabia Project (TESS) project demonstrated teleconsultation was feasible to improve stroke care in rural areas where management in a stroke unit is hindered by long transportation distances [65]. Similar to the virtual stroke unit, tele-neurocritical care units are safe, reliable, cost-saving strategies that improve the timely response to neurologic ICU emergencies, decrease hospital lengths of stay, and improve functional outcomes [117].

Inpatient neurology has also observed an increase in need for stroke care despite a shortage of vascular neurologists. This interactive videoconferencing in which patients, caregivers, and providers can all interact at the bedside and remotely communicate in real time is a huge shift from the more historical methods patient care. Vascular neurohospitalists can also use telemedicine to meet demand, adding another dimension to quality inpatient care [118,119]. A remote specialist can also advise regarding a patient's care via inpatient teleneurology. In all models, network hospitals must have specific agreements and protocols to transfer patients with stroke or thrombolysis complications [30]. Telestroke services for inpatients require the same oversight as emergency telestroke programs. Additional personnel, including rapid response teams and other emergency responders, would be included in these reviews to ensure appropriate metrics are met. Opportunities also exist for telestroke to be used to identify and enroll patients in clinical trials of acute stroke treatment. These technical advances significantly extend the foundation on which telestroke can be built (Table 2.4).

Table 2.4 Telestroke terms and definitions.

Distant Site—Telestroke provider location; sometimes used interchangeably with hub site when referencing a hub and spoke network.

Distributed Network—A model in which telestroke services are provided to multiple originating sites through arrangements with an independent corporation or an affiliated network of telestroke providers. In this setting, transfer agreements for endovascular therapy or subsequent stroke care should be defined in advance to facilitate all aspects of acute stroke care.

Hub—Typically a comprehensive tertiary care center where vascular neurologists and other acute stroke specialists compose a call panel delivering telestroke services to network affiliate/partner sites—spokes. If a patient requires transfer to a higher level of care, a hub is usually the destination. Some networks may have multiple hubs.

Hub and Spoke—Networks of primary, secondary, and tertiary care settings that provide care to specific patient populations. Networks may vary in

Table 2.4 Telestroke terms and definitions.—cont'd

sophistication, with many working as loose coalitions of segregated services. Typically, specialty care is provided to patients at remote settings (often rural emergency departments [EDs]) by specialists affiliated with larger, more comprehensive tertiary care centers. Models are changing with an emphasis on keeping patients in their local community when possible, depending on the available level of care.

m-Health—Mobile health.

Originating Site—Patient location; sometimes used interchangeably with spoke site when referencing a hub and spoke network model.

Spoke—The affiliate or partner site in a telestroke network, underserviced or under supported by neurologists, where patient services are delivered.

Teleconsent—A telemedicine-based approach to obtaining informed consent and offers a unique solution to limitations of traditional consent approaches.

Teleneurology—Broad application of telemedicine to the field of neurology, both acute and ambulatory care.

Teleneurohospitalist—A neurohospitalist who provides teleneurology services to an ED and/or a hospital located remote to their immediate geographic physical practice.

Teleneurologic intensive care unit (teleneuro-ICU)—Provides continuous intensive care unit (ICU) monitoring and consultation from an intensivist at a remote location.

Telestroke—A network of audiovisual communication and computer systems, which provide the foundation for a collaborative, interprofessional care model focusing on acute stroke patients. Focus is on the evaluation of patients with acute stroke syndromes for possible intravenous recombinant tissue plasminogen activator (IV rtPA) administration or other emergency stroke treatments. Telestroke has developed rapidly and has accumulated a large body of evidence-based literature supporting its use in evaluating patients with stroke remotely.

Telestroke Network—A group of primary, secondary, and tertiary care settings that provide acute stroke care to their patient population. Telestroke networks consist of originating sites where the patients are located and distant sites where the telestroke provider is situated. Telestroke systems exist either as a distributed or a hub and spoke model.

Telestrokologist—A strokologist who is proficient with telemedicine tools and techniques necessary for remote stroke practice.

Adapted from Demaerschalk BM, et al. American telemedicine association: telestroke guidelines. Telemed J Health 2017;23(5):376—389.

CHAPTER 3

Telestroke examination

Current stroke guidelines emphasize the value of telestroke to support the immediate assessment of stroke severity via the National Institutes of Health Stroke Scale (NIHSS) and other instruments and its equivalence to that of a bedside assessment. Over the past several years, the remote evaluation of stroke patients has been validated in the prehospital setting particularly in mobile stroke units, emergency department, and inpatient stroke units (including assessments of occupational, physical, or speech disability in stroke patients by allied health professionals). In the wake of the COVID-19 pandemic, nonacute stroke evaluation has also been utilized in the outpatient setting to protect patients and staff and limit viral spread.

Data on the feasibility and reliability of conducting a general neurological evaluation over telemedicine compared well with face-to-face consultation [322]. Modifications of the telemedicine neurologic examination are necessary to have a successful stroke evaluation [323–325]. Stroke severity scales can be reliably administered via telemedicine for both acute and subacute stroke patients and the items with the highest interrater reliability generally include level of consciousness and motor-related questions. Items with the lowest interrater reliability generally include facial palsy, ataxia, and dysarthria. These findings are similar to bedside reliability assessments [29,58,105].

For the hyperacute/acute stroke evaluation, the NIHSS assessment tool is recommended. This is designed to measure the neurologic deficits most often seen with acute stroke patients. It is a nonlinear ordinal scale, with possible scores ranging from 0 to 42. In-person exam performance has been timed to take 5–8 min with slightly longer assessments (mean 9.70 versus 6.55 min, $P < 001$) for the remote evaluation [29]. For the NIHSS-telestroke assessment, high-quality video teleconference (HQ-VTC) closely matches with NIHSS-bedside assessment. Interrater agreement for the NIHSS demonstrated a reliable assessment. Based on weighted kappa coefficients, four items (orientation, motor arm, motor leg, and neglect) displayed excellent agreement, six items (language, dysarthria, sensation, visual fields, facial palsy, and gaze) displayed good agreement, and two items

TeleStroke
ISBN 978-0-12-824161-5
https://doi.org/10.1016/B978-0-12-824161-5.00003-7
© 2021 Elsevier Inc.
All rights reserved.

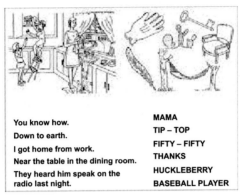

You know how. Down to earth. I got home from work. Near the table in the dining room. They heard him speak on the radio last night.	MAMA TIP – TOP FIFTY – FIFTY THANKS HUCKLEBERRY BASEBALL PLAYER

Figure 3.1 Pictures of NIHSS.

(commands and ataxia) displayed poor agreement. Total NIHSS scores obtained by bedside and remote methods were strongly correlated ($r = 0.97$, $P < .001$) [326].

For the evaluation assess orientation (How old are you?, what month is it?). Assess the ability to describe the picture and to read standardized sentences. Assess visual fields and inattention in four quadrants. Assess the pupillary light reflex and eye movements following the "H" pattern. Assess facial sensation (may be more difficult if no one to assist). Assess facial movements (have patient close eyes, smile) (Fig. 3.1).

Outpatient evaluation

For the outpatient evaluations, it is important to set expectations and ask patients to have key items such as pen and paper, flashlight, thermometer, and blood pressure cuff. It is recommended that a family member be present during the appointment to assist with the examination process. It is important that the assessment be performed through a secure online platform that is compliant with local privacy acts and your compliance team policies. The patient should be asked to verify their identity by providing their address or date of birth or showing photographic identification. Verbal consent to perform the remote evaluation must be obtained and documented. Standard language can be integrated into your note or electronic health record (EHR). The American Telemedicine Association has sample consent forms. One example provided on the website: "This is a telemedicine visit that was performed with the originating site at [INSERT PATIENT LOCATION] and the distant site at [INSERT PROVIDER

LOCATION]. Verbal consent to participate in video visit was obtained. This visit occurred during the Coronavirus (COVID-19) Public Health Emergency. I discussed with the patient the nature of our telemedicine visits, that: • I would evaluate the patient and recommend diagnostics and treatments based on my assessment • Our sessions are not being recorded and that personal health information is protected • Our team would provide follow up care in person if/when the patient needs it" [327].

If required, a translator should be present (either a family member or formal third-party translation services). Maintaining eye contact and being attentive during the evaluation is important. If you need to view another screen during the evaluation, explain to the patient why you are looking away. The virtual examination should be performed without visual obstructions between the patient and camera. The room should allow for privacy, be well lit, and open with room for the patient to move closer or farther from the camera during the examination and enough space to observe gait.

General assessment and vitals

General appearance can be made by inspection during the video visit. The patient can use home equipment such as thermometer and blood pressure cuff to check temperature, blood pressure, and pulse.

Neurological examination (modified from Ref. [322])

Mental status and cognitive testing

For patients with visual, auditory, and/or cognitive deficits some elements of this examination may be observational only.

1. For a basic cognitive evaluation, orientation can be examined by assessing place (city) and time (day, date, month, and year).
2. The patient should be asked to look directly at the camera while answering orientation questions so as to avoid the use of environmental cues (phones, calendars, watches).
3. To test attention, instruct the patient to state the months of the year backward or subtract backward from 100 by 7's.
4. Evaluate comprehension by assessing midline commands, appendicular commands, and cross midline commands.
5. Naming, fluency and recent episodic memory, presence of phonemic or semantic paraphasic errors, or the presence of apraxia of speech can all be assessed.

6. Test naming of high frequency and low-frequency words and assess repetition by having the patient repeat a sentence such as "no ifs ands or buts."

7. Then ask the patient to follow simple commands to test comprehension, such as "close your eyes" and more complex tasks such as "point to the ceiling and then the floor."

8. An expanded cognitive assessment may be performed such as the Montreal Cognitive Assessment and the Mini-Mental State Examination. However, patients will need a pen and paper and may need to print out the necessary images. Most telemedicine software allows for screen sharing and whiteboard use, which is helpful to share any relevant images.

Cranial nerve examination

The patient will need to be close to the camera in order to assess the rest of the cranial nerve exam by assessing pupils, tongue, and jaw movements. Formal visual acuity assessment cannot be reliably performed through video. There have been many advances in camera technology, intelligent software, and cloud computing paradigms but it is still difficult to reliably perform this via video [328]. If using cards, these should be well illuminated.

1. Examiners can ask the patient to cover one eye at a time and ask them what they see, using a red object to assess red desaturation or use the NIH stroke scale cards to test for visual field defects. If assessment of vision is critical, the patient can be referred to a recognized website that provides printable Snellen charts.

2. Ask the patient to position their face about 2 feet away from the monitor while looking at an object held by the examiner (e.g., pen) and then ask the patient if they can see all four corners of the monitor may allow the examiner to screen for a gross field cut (such as a marked hemianopia).

3. Pupillary constriction can be assessed by having the patient cover one eye and then uncover, followed by the other eye and watching for the appropriate response. With the patient's face centered and close to the camera, observe for pupillary asymmetry, ptosis, ocular alignment, or abnormal eye movements such as nystagmus.

4. To test ocular motility, ask the patient to look in the nine cardinal positions of gaze, and it may be necessary to ask the patient to manually lift their eyelids during downgaze. Ask the patient to briefly pause at each gaze position looking for nystagmus.

5. Horizontal saccades can be tested by asking the patient to alternate their gaze between the top right and left corners of the computer screen.
6. Vertical saccades can be tested by asking the patient to alternate their gaze between just above the computer monitor and just below it.
7. Inspect for temporalis atrophy and ask the patient to open their mouth, looking for jaw deviation.
8. If concern for facial sensory disturbance, the patient can check sensation over the sensory distributions of the trigeminal nerve side-to-side with a tissue or something cold (e.g., ice pack).
9. Observe baseline facial symmetry, including reduced movement on one side of the face and flattening of the nasolabial fold.
10. Ask the patient to raise their eyebrows, close their eyes tight, purse their lips, show their teeth, and puff out their cheeks.
11. Hearing cannot be formally assessed, and unilateral hearing loss cannot be confirmed through video.
12. Ask the patient to phonate ("pa," "ta," and "ka"). Depending on video quality and lighting, ask the patient to open their mouth and observe soft palate elevation.
13. Ask the patient to expose the neck and shoulders, evaluating for atrophy of the sternocleidomastoid and trapezius muscles. Have the patient look to the right and then the left and then to shrug their shoulders to test muscle activation.
14. Depending on video quality, observe the tongue in the mouth, looking for fasciculations or atrophy. Ask the patient to protrude the tongue, and move the tongue side to side rapidly.

Motor examination

1. Assesses pronator drift, leg drift, and coordination and gait similarly to an in-person evaluation. Nonconfrontational measures to assess upper extremity strength using pronator/Digit Quinti sign/Barrel roll/finger taps for subtle signs of weakness.
2. For the lower limbs, position the camera downward. While seated, ask the patient to raise each knee off the chair, to straighten the knees one at a time, and to dorsiflex and then plantarflex each foot. With arms crossed across the chest, ask them to stand up. The patient can be asked to do 1—10 squats, to assess for fatigability or subtle proximal leg weakness. The patient should be asked to perform heel raises (dorsiflexion strength), and then do single foot toe raises (plantarflexion strength). They can also be asked to stand and hop on each leg.

3. Axial muscle strength can be tested by asking the patient to perform sit-ups.
4. Tone, reflexes, and plantar responses cannot be formally assessed.
5. Observe the patient with the arms at rest and then raise for abnormal movements (tremor, myoclonus, chorea, dystonia, or others).
6. Subtle signs of pyramidal weakness can be detected by assessing for pronator drift, using the forearm rolling test, and testing of fine finger movements (tapping thumb with index finger repetitively or with each finger alternatively).

Sensory examination

This is more subjective; an onsite assistant may improve assessment. For a basic evaluation, one could ask the patient to use an ice pack or cooled spoon to compare light touch or temperature on the index fingers of both hands and the top of the big toes. Assess sensory ataxia by asking the patient can raise their arms, close their eyes, and touch their nose with each index finger separately.

Coordination

1. If onsite assistant is present, they can be asked to hold their finger out for standard finger-to-nose testing. If unavailable, ask the patient to hold an object (such as a pen) outstretched in front of them with one hand, and then with the contralateral index finger perform finger-to-object movements and then repeat on the contralateral side.
2. Alternatively, the patient can be asked to hold their arms outstretched in front of them, and then touch their nose with each index finger.
3. Rapid alternating movements can be checked as usual.
4. Bradykinesia testing can be performed by having the patient perform finger taps and palm opening and closing maneuvers in both arms observing for any fatigability.
5. Heel-to-shin testing can be performed by asking the patient to put each leg on a stool or ottoman and performing the maneuver.
6. The patient can also be asked to perform foot tapping and heel stomping.

Gait

There may be limitations based on camera setup or size of the room. Observe stance at rest and with the feet together.

1. Ask the patient to walk in two directions from one side of the room to the other and then walk away from the camera, turn around, and walk back to the camera.
2. Ask the patient to attempt five steps in either direction before turning around.
3. Tandem gait can be assessed similarly. It is not recommended to perform the Romberg test given the risk of the patient falling without the examiner to catch them.

CHAPTER 4

Telehealth initiation and expansion during COVID-19 global pandemic

In December 2019, the first case of the novel coronavirus COVID-19 was identified in China. On March 11, 2020, the World Health Organization declared the coronavirus disease 2019 (COVID-19) a pandemic, and in the weeks following, public health organizations, medical associations, and governing bodies throughout the world recommended limiting contact with others to "flatten the curve" of COVID-19. Several countries including the United States implemented stay-at-home orders. Hospitals canceled elective procedures and outpatient in-person clinic visits to minimize the exposure risk to patients and healthcare workers. The landscape of stroke telehealth and limitations of strained health systems was challenged to establish and rapidly deploy telehealth services to meet the needs of their community. Yet, to meet these challenges, health systems had to maintain safe practices with severely limited resources.

The COVID-19 pandemic led to dramatic changes in healthcare delivery and offered a unique opportunity to innovate and expand telestroke limits not only during this crisis but in anticipation of other disasters. It brought a compelling opportunity to leverage novel technological platforms to transform telehealth. Widespread implementation of telehealth during the COVID-19 pandemic led to transformational changes in policies with expanded coverage, reimbursement parity for in-person and remote visits and legislative changes [120,121]. Medicare temporarily expanded its coverage of telemedicine to all beneficiaries, included in-home visits and paid for audio-only visits at the same rate as video and in-person visits. In addition, rapid modification of inpatient and emergency department pathways was necessary to reduce the risk of COVID-19 exposure, protect healthcare providers, and preserve personal protective equipment (PPE) supplies while maintaining the need for a rapid and comprehensive assessment [122,123].

In January 2020 after the declaration of a COVID-19 public health emergency, there were near-daily changes that impacted a practice or hospital's finances. CMS made changes to reimbursement to make it easier

TeleStroke
ISBN 978-0-12-824161-5
https://doi.org/10.1016/B978-0-12-824161-5.00004-9

© 2021 Elsevier Inc.
All rights reserved.

for people enrolled in Medicare, Medicaid, and the Children's Health Insurance Program (CHIP) to receive medical care through telehealth services during the COVID-19 Public Health Emergency. States temporarily waived licensure requirements. Payment parity policies were also implemented. Each state's Medicaid program varies on the use of telehealth. Some states have very expansive telehealth policies, and other states are rapidly expanding their allowance of telehealth to monitor and treat COVID-19. These significant changes allowed providers to conduct telehealth with patients located in their homes and outside of designated rural areas; practice remote care, even across state lines, through telehealth, deliver care to both established and new patients through telehealth, bill for telehealth services (both video and audio-only) as if they were provided in person [121,124,125]. CMS significantly expanded the list of covered telehealth services that can be provided in Medicare to include emergency department visits, initial nursing facility and discharge visits, home visits and therapy services [121]. Whether this will lead to a permanent shift in telehealth services is unknown.

To examine changes in the frequency of use of telehealth services during the early pandemic period, the CDC analyzed deidentified encounter (i.e., visit) data from four of the largest US telehealth providers that offer services in all states. Trends in telehealth encounters during January—March 2020 (surveillance weeks 1—13) were compared with encounters occurring during the same weeks in 2019. Telehealth visits during this time increased by 50% compared to the same period in 2019 [126].

In March 2020, the Office of Civil Rights (OCR) within the Department of Health and Human Services (HHS) relaxed its enforcement of HIPAA rules during the COVID-19 public health emergency. OCR exercised its enforcement discretion and would not impose penalties for noncompliance with the regulatory requirements under the HIPAA Rules against covered healthcare providers in connection with the good faith provision of telehealth during the COVID-19 nationwide public health emergency. As a result, a covered healthcare provider using audio—video communication technology to provide telehealth to patients during the COVID-19 nationwide public health emergency can use any nonpublic facing remote communication product that is available to communicate with patients [121]. As such, widely available apps such as FaceTime and Skype could be used in good faith for any telehealth treatment or diagnostic purpose, regardless of whether the telehealth service is directly related to COVID-19.

The American Stroke Association provided emergency guidance for overall hyperacute treatment of stroke and recommended individual institutions devise emergency care pathways that provide systematic guidance to all members of the stroke team [120]. Finding the right balance when adjusting guidelines and stroke pathways to maintain high quality of care and minimize the chances of contributing to the rapid spread of COVID-19 was challenging. Telestroke allowed patients to be evaluated at spoke site hospitals and prevented unnecessary transfers. Hyperacute telestroke evaluations reduced exposure for clinicians and preserved the scarce supply of PPE.

This model from researchers at the University of California, San Diego (UCSD), highlights the modifications created to adapt the workflow during the pandemic from their standard protocol. All patients undergo COVID screening. The adapted UCSD model also provides for in-person assessment if telestroke systems are not available for any reason (e.g., power outage, Internet access outage, telestroke software failure, etc.) [116]. COVID-19 is known to have a high rate of fomite transmission [127,128]. Cleaning protocols for devices were established by several institutions and telemedicine device companies to reduce contamination. Providers are encouraged to avoid the use of hospital-based phones and computers unless properly cleaned. Personal devices enabled with dual authentication applications used for phone calls, texting/paging, and EHR documentation should be cleaned often in the hospital and upon leaving [116]. Similarly, use of imaging modalities such as magnetic resonance image (MRI) was obtained only if it would change the treatment recommendations, as the cleaning protocol would require hours before next use. This allowed reduced risk of transmission to imaging and transport personnel. The additional protective measures also impacted infection control in ambulances, MSUs, and neuro-angiography suites. The University of Cincinnati and the Society of Vascular and Interventional Neurology provided concrete guidance on how to minimize delays to EVT while keeping the risk of infectious exposure for patients and staff at a minimum [129,130]. (See Figs. 4.1 and 4.2).

Although both ischemic and hemorrhagic strokes have been reported with COVID-19, there was early anecdotal suggestion of an overall decrease in stroke admissions. A Mayo Clinic study reported "a clinically important reduction in telestroke activations was seen in the 30 days following the WHO declaration of the COVID-19 pandemic. This reduction mirrors early data regarding reduction of ST-segment elevation

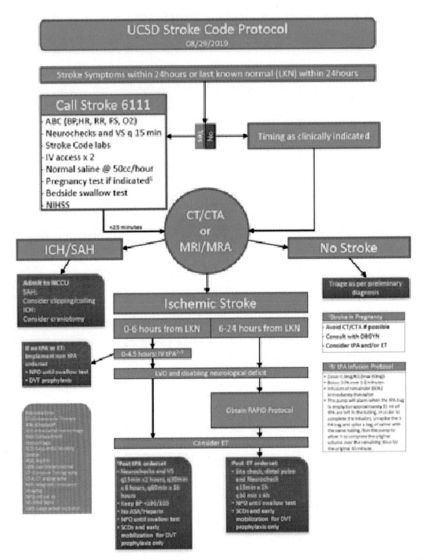

Figure 4.1 The stroke code protocol per University of California San Diego Medical Center Policy to optimize stroke treatment and outcomes [116].

myocardial infarction as well as single-center reports of reduced stroke volumes and interventions globally" [131]. Similar findings were noted in Connecticut, where hospital presentation for stroke-like symptoms decreased without differences in stroke severity or early outcomes [132]. Shah et al. observed a significant and rapid decline in telestroke consults and

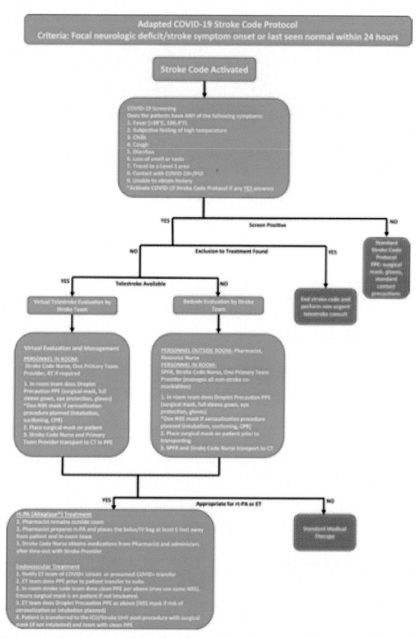

Figure 4.2 The adapted COVID-19 UCSD stroke code protocol focuses on the rapid assessment of stroke code patients that may be eligible for thrombolysis and/or endovascular treatment. The use of PPE is reduced by either telestroke consultation or reduced personnel required to be physically in-room [116].

postulated that fear of contracting coronavirus, social distancing, and isolation likely played a major role in the reduction [133]. The COVID-19 pandemic has been disruptive for acute telestroke pathways. It is critical to encourage patients to continue seeking emergency care if experiencing acute stroke symptoms. It is also vital to avoid breaks in the stroke chain of survival by encouraging providers to use stroke code activation and telestroke networks.

CHAPTER 5

Hyperacute telestroke

Stroke patients who reach the hospital within 1 h of symptoms receive a clot-busting drug twice as often as those arriving later. Researchers call the first hour of symptom onset "the golden hour." Among more than 100,000 patients treated at hospitals participating in the American Heart Association's Get With The Guidelines—Stroke (GWTG—Stroke) quality improvement program, 27.1% who arrived within the "golden hour" were treated with tissue plasminogen activator (tPA). Jeffrey Saver demonstrated for every minute in which a stroke is untreated, the average patient loses 1.9 million neurons, 13.8 billion synapses, and seven miles of axonal fibers. With each hour in which treatment fails to occur, the brain loses as many neurons as it does in almost 3.6 years of normal aging [162]. Acute ischemic stroke is an emergency and requires effective triage, diagnosis, and critical management. The hyperacute management of ischemic stroke begins in the field, with recognition of stroke symptoms by emergency medical systems (EMSs) personnel. A proficient stroke system of care uses diagnostic algorithms for EMS activation and response. These systematically evaluate each potential acute stroke patient, provide appropriate emergent care to each patient, and transport each patient to the most appropriate hospital. EMS providers are responsible to obtain as accurate a patient history as possible, including establishing the last known well time, or time of stroke symptom onset. This information is essential in determining whether an acute stroke patient is a candidate to receive intravenous thrombolysis [163].

The model of "hub-and-spoke" comprises a central institution (primary stroke center (PSC) or comprehensive stroke center (CSC)) which acts as a hub to remote hospitals (spoke) with whom they are contracted to provide telestroke. Stroke neurologists at the hub supervise the evaluation and management of acute stroke patients at spokes via telestroke (more often with video consultation although telephone can be used). If patients are determined to be appropriate intravenous tPA candidates, it will be initiated at the spoke hospital. If indicated, the patient can then be transferred to the hub hospital ("drip and ship"). Telestroke is safe and feasible and clinical outcomes between hospitals utilizing telestroke and PSCs, including mortality, are similar. The comprehensive benefit from telestroke networks

TeleStroke
ISBN 978-0-12-824161-5
https://doi.org/10.1016/B978-0-12-824161-5.00005-0

© 2021 Elsevier Inc.
All rights reserved.

on improved functional outcome have not been demonstrated in a randomized controlled trial. However, there are several studies which have demonstrated a positive effect on thrombolysis rates and functional outcomes of acute stroke patients [86,89]. Stroke patients from community hospitals with telemedical support within the Telemedical Project for Integrative Stroke Care (TEMPiS) were more likely to receive IV thrombolysis and less likely to have a poor functional outcome at 3 months compared to matched stroke patients from community hospitals without specialized stroke care [86]. Mortality and symptomatic intracranial hemorrhage (sICH) rates did not differ significantly among patients treated in Telestroke networks or in tertiary care stroke centers in these studies, thus indicating the safety of the telemedical approach [27,86,89,104].

For vascular neurology, remote consultation has significantly improved access to care for patients presenting with symptoms of acute stroke or transient ischemic attack. Telestroke has quickly spread throughout the United States, with at least 56 networks in 27 states linking a stroke center with local hospitals that lack around the clock stroke expertise [158]. In addition to safety and improved rates of thrombolysis, telestroke has also been demonstrated to improve stroke outcomes. The increased use of tPA with telestroke has led to direct comparisons of clinical outcomes in networked and out of network hospitals. In a prospective study comparing 3 month outcomes after an AIS in 3122 cases, the composite outcome of death, institutionalization, or disability was significantly less likely in telestroke hospitals than comparable out of network hospitals (44% and 54%, respectively) [30,31,164]. Audebert et al. via multivariate regression analysis showed that presentation to a telestroke hospital was independently associated with a reduced risk of a poor outcome [164]. Remote consultation led to higher rates of diagnostic and therapeutic interventions in cases of AIS, with at least 75% of consultations resulting in a meaningful change in management [65].

In an effort to increase access to stroke care, some health systems are using mobile stroke units (MSUs). The MSU is an ambulance unit with onboard CT-scanning technology and a specialist team who can provide treatment onsite and decide if advanced treatment is required. Having imaging capacity can expedite stroke diagnosis and treatment. Studies have demonstrated that remote reading of head CT imaging by a critical care physician on an MSU was found to have excellent agreement with hospital radiologists in identifying candidates for prehospital thrombolysis [165]. In Australia and Berlin, MSUs have demonstrated improvements in metropolitan alarm-to-treatment time. Studies have demonstrated a significant reduction in treatment delays compared to standard emergency department admissions, with almost 50% of patients being treated within the "golden hour" One of the first European MSUs saw a 10-fold rise in successful "golden-hour" treatments when compared to conventional treatment [166–170]. However, the MSU is limited by distance and usually operates within a 20 km radius from the base hospital to ensure "golden hour" treatment. This makes it challenging for less urban communities to rapidly access treatment.

MSUs can be difficult to staff, and are expensive to implement. In the United States, prehospital stroke treatment is unlikely to be cost-effective if a physician must be onboard [171]. MSUs have been deployed since May 2014. These units are generally staffed 100% of the time with a paramedic, CT technologist, a registered nurse experienced in managing acute stroke patients, and a vascular neurologist either in person or remote. The BEST-MSU study (Benefits of Stroke Treatment Delivered Using a Mobile Stroke Unit) will help to determine if remote vascular neurology assessment is comparable to onboard and thus help assess cost effectiveness [172,173]. An Ohio pilot study of the MSU solely using telemedicine for virtual vascular neurologist and neuro-radiologist support virtually demonstrated a significant decrease in time-to-treatment compared to a control group brought to the emergency department via ambulance [174]. The ability to identify ischemic stroke in the field may also expedite patient transfer to thrombectomy-capable facility, reducing overall transfer time (See Fig. 5.1).

In MSU-based stroke management, patients are diagnosed at the site of emergency, allowing case-specific treatment and triage to the most appropriate stroke center, thus avoiding secondary transfers. In conventional stroke management, due to insufficient knowledge about the cause of

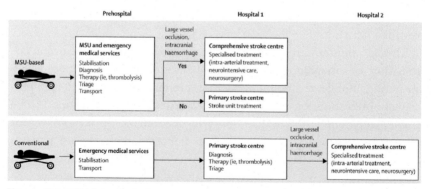

Figure 5.1 MSU-based stroke management compared with conventional stroke management.

the symptoms, patients are transported to the PSC and eventually, by secondary transfer, brought to a CSC [175].

In select patients with emergent large vessel occlusions, endovascular management improves functional outcomes and mortality [176–178]. As with IV thrombolysis, remote and underserved communities have limited access to endovascular therapy (EVT) but lack of access is also seen in urban areas [179,180]. It is important to accurately identify potential EVT candidates and prompt video assessment can facilitate evaluation. Current guidelines recommend consideration of EVT for NIHSS score greater than 6 as this may be predictive of a large vessel occlusion [66]. Rapid assessment and decision to transfer helps avoid transfer delays which can limit the use of EVT in acute stroke. Telestroke provides effective triage of patients likely to benefit from more EVT. It allows for remote consent through video interface for EVT in advance, reducing delays in proceeding with thrombectomy once the patient arrives at the hub [181]. This has been demonstrated in a Spanish telestroke network where remote assessment facilitated prompt thrombolysis and transfer for endovascular management of AIS [182]. In this "drip, ship, and retrieve" model, informed consent was obtained remotely and the angiography suite was prepared while the patient was en route, facilitating faster groin puncture times in telestroke versus out of network transfers. Three months postinfarct, functional outcomes were comparable between patients initially treated at the referral center or via telestroke, but significantly worse in patients in out of network facilities [30,182]. Barlinn et al. in a retrospective observational study demonstrated that telestroke networks may enable delivery of EVT to selected ischemic stroke patients transferred from remote hospitals that is equitable to patients admitted directly to tertiary hospitals [183]. The study highlighted the need to implement time- and quality-driven algorithms for identification, transfer, and initiation of EVT into existing telestroke networks (See Fig. 5.2).

Mobile communication systems can provide seamless concurrent coordination of emergent stroke care and decision-making support [184]. Integrating mobile technologies such as prehospital assessment and prehospital notification for AIS into the EMS system has been reported to be feasible and beneficial [185]. The Field Assessment Stroke Triage for Emergency Destination (FAST-ED) app improves the triage of patients with AIS, reduces hospital arrivals times, and maximizes the use of thrombolytic therapy [185]. There are also widely used free mobile applications, such as WhatsApp [186]. However, some have raised concern that some of these apps may not be HIPAA-compliant for use in a

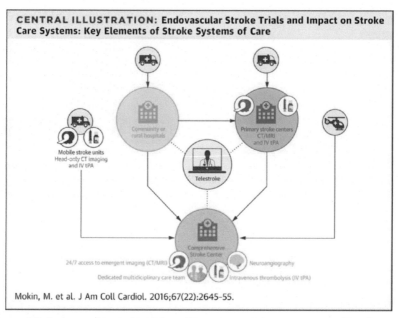

Figure 5.2 Endovascular stroke trials and impact on stroke care systems: Key elements of stroke systems of care.

healthcare setting [187]. There are also several applications built to assist with physical findings on the neurological exam (e.g., iPronator) and to assist in calculating and tracking National Institutes of Health Stroke Scale (NeuroToolkit, Medequations) [188]. In recent years, automated stroke diagnostic tools integrating both clinical and radiological data have fostered growth in teleradiology for acute stroke care. Viewing neuroimaging remotely has become feasible and practical for emergent scenarios on mobile devices. Tablet-based radiology platforms have been shown to expedite preliminary imaging interpretations in acute stroke management. For example, the "i-Stroke" system was developed to transfer clinical data, computed tomography (CT), magnetic resonance imaging (MRI), angiographic and intraoperative images, as well as expert opinion, all in real time [189]. Validation studies have shown high sensitivity and specificity, as well as high intraobserver reliability, for ischemic stroke and large vessel occlusions, when viewed on mobile device [159,165]. (See Fig. 5.3).

A CSC provides the highest level of care for acute stroke patients and has 24/7 access to emergent imaging (CT/MRI), intravenous [IV] thrombolysis, and neuroangiography, and a dedicated multidisciplinary

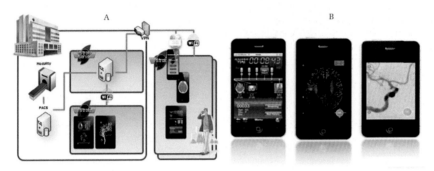

Figure 5.3 (A) Components of the system (SYNAPSE Erm) for connecting off- and on-site medical care providers. (B) Display of the diagnostic and treatment data on mobile devices [190].

team (stroke neurology, neurointerventional, neurosurgery, and neuro-critical care teams). CSCs can accept patients directly or via interhospital transfer from PSCs (which can administer IV thrombolysis) or from community or rural hospitals. Telestroke works closely with CSCs and other hospitals to determine which patients require IV thrombolysis, endovascular thrombectomy, or both. MSUs allow administration of IV thrombolysis "in the field," with potential for bypass of PSCs and transfer of those patients who are candidates for endovascular therapy directly to CSCs. NICU = neurointensive care unit; rtPA = recombinant tissue plasminogen activator; tPA = tissue plasminogen activator [191].

CHAPTER 6

Pediatric telestroke

Pediatric emergency department visits account for approximately 20% of all emergency department visits [258]. However, fewer than 7% of emergency departments in the United States have all the necessary supplies for managing pediatric emergencies or enough trained pediatric emergency personnel [139,259,260]. When compared with no consultations, pediatric telemedicine in rural emergency departments demonstrated higher physician-rated quality of care, higher patient satisfaction, and lower risk of physician-related medication errors [261—264]. Brova et al. found only 8% of US emergency departments currently utilize pediatric telemedicine and of the sampled emergency departments equipped with telemedicine technology, the equipment was seldomly used [264]. Interestingly, most of the emergency departments using pediatric telemedicine were not staffed by board-certified or board-eligible pediatric emergency medicine physicians or pediatricians [264]. In 2012, the Institute of Medicine endorsed the role of pediatric emergency telemedicine in the US healthcare system [265]. In 2015, the American Academy of Pediatrics issued a policy statement on the expanding role of telehealth in pediatrics to highlight the ability of this technology to improve aspects of pediatric care and help deal with workforce shortages [266]. Yet, despite these recommendations, pediatric telemedicine in the emergency setting remains relatively underutilized compared with ambulatory telemedicine [153,267—269].

Pediatric telemedicine has been used in various outpatient specialties including genetics, cardiology, dermatology, psychiatry, and surgery [270—277]. The technology can be used in the inpatient (emergency or intensive unit), ambulatory, and home setting. Neurologists can perform inpatient consults for specific disease populations such as epilepsy, stroke, and movement disorders for example in a community hospital without access to neurologic expertise. In the ambulatory and home setting, they can provide follow-up care for stroke, headache, epilepsy, and neurodevelopmental disabilities among others [99,100,278—280]. These visits can also focus on counseling, education, and reviewing diagnostic test results. They are useful in situations when the patient is unable to leave the home or when it is challenging for the family to get to an ambulatory clinic [100]. Pediatric care

TeleStroke
ISBN 978-0-12-824161-5
https://doi.org/10.1016/B978-0-12-824161-5.00006-2

© 2021 Elsevier Inc.
All rights reserved.

involves the participation of family members and other individuals, such as teachers, therapists, psychologists, and even primary care providers. It is important to obtain all relevant information from each depending on the acuity of the evaluation. In addition, during the COVID-19 pandemic, rapid implementation of telemedicine in a large pediatric neurology network demonstrated that it was feasible and effective for a large proportion of this patient population [278]. Outcome studies demonstrate pediatric telemedicine has an impact on parent satisfaction, reduced absenteeism due to illness, reduced travel time and costs, reduced emergency department use for nonurgent conditions, and reduction in fragmentation of care by patients seeking services at urgent care clinics [281—285].

Pediatric stroke occurs in 1.2—2.4 per 100 000 children/y in developed countries [286—288]. In the United States, cerebrovascular disease is among the top 10 causes of pediatric mortality and pediatric stroke survivors face decades of living with disability [289]. There are no clinical trials to guide the emergency treatment of acute pediatric acute ischemic stroke. Literature regarding management of pediatric stroke including the use of antithrombotic therapy, the role of thrombolytics, and endovascular therapy for children is sparse with conflicting evidence [187,290]. Early recognition and evaluation of acute stroke symptoms in children has increased in the last decade with several institutions developing pediatric acute stroke pathways. The Thrombolysis in Pediatric Stroke trial encouraged pediatric stroke centers to have designated stroke teams, imaging protocols, and pathways for rapid assessment and identification of children with stroke. This increase in preparedness can identify children as candidates for tPA and thrombectomy [291—293]. However, there is limited data regarding the use of telestroke in pediatric populations.

Pediatric telestroke allows pediatric subspecialists and vascular neurologists the opportunity to provide expertise to children needing acute and chronic stroke care. Building on these models, telehealth technology not only benefits children in urban and rural medically underserved regions but also has the potential to reduce socioeconomic disparities and improve the quality of pediatric emergency stroke care in underserved areas [139,153,262,263,268,269,294]. Lack of access to specialty care, late arrivals to appointments, or missed appointments due to long distances are significant challenges faced by families. Pediatric telestroke can diminish parent frustration, provide stroke specific expertise, and overall improve patient care [100]. Health systems with ready access to pediatric subspecialty care may also benefit from telemedicine particularly in teaching hospitals with

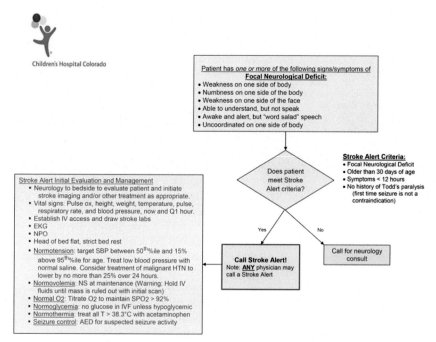

Children's Hospital Colorado

Figure 6.1 Pediatric code stroke protocol [291].

residents and fellow as it provides real-time attending supervision and oversight of complex cases [295]. (See Fig. 6.1).

There are many challenges with pediatric telestroke care in the United States. This includes differentiating acute ischemic stroke from stroke mimics such as migraine, conversion disorders, and seizures which can be seen in 21%—76% of pediatric patients undergoing evaluation for acute neurological symptoms [296,297]. Delayed pediatric acute ischemic stroke diagnosis can also occur as a result of delay in stroke recognition. Studies have reported that parents often do not consider stroke as a diagnosis when their child has stroke-like symptoms [298—300]. An Australian study found 83% of parents thought immediate actions were required when their children developed neurological symptoms; however, less than half of them considered stroke as a possibility [301]. Almost one-quarter waited to see whether symptoms would resolve before seeking medical attention [301]. (See Table 6.1).

Adult stroke recognition tools such as the Los Angeles Prehospital Stroke Screen can improve diagnostic accuracy in the prehospital and ED settings by selecting elements of the neurological examination with the highest reliability for stroke diagnosis [287,302]. However, use of adult

Table 6.1 Potential challenges with acute pediatric telestroke evaluations.

Challenges	Potential solutions
Prehospital recognition of possible stroke, delays in arrival to hospital	• Public awareness and education campaigns regarding childhood stroke • Develop decision support tools to improve EMS recognition of stroke • Improve pediatric stroke awareness in the medical community (subspecialty physicians who care for children with high risk of stroke)
Clinical differentiation of stroke versus mimics	• Develop decision support tools to improve pediatric ED physician recognition of stroke • Education regarding differential of acute neurological symptoms in children • Development of Pediatric Code Stroke Alert
Pediatric tools for stroke assessment	• Utilize the pediatric NIHSS if possible • Development of pediatric acute stroke pathways and systems approach to care
Accessing rapid diagnostic imaging	• CT scans can lead to diagnostic delays, set up acute stroke neuroimaging pathways to obtain rapid MRI • Develop process for anesthesia/sedation
Safety and efficacy of thrombolysis/thrombectomy in children	• Need for more prospective studies in children • Establish pediatric registries to capture safety and efficacy data for reperfusion therapies • Thoughtful consideration of treatment options on a case-by-case basis using a team-based approach with pediatric team, stroke specialist, neurointerventionalist • Improve access to centers with experience in endovascular therapies in children, develop rapid transfer pathways

Adapted from Lehman LL, et al. What will improve pediatric acute stroke care? Stroke 2019;50(2):249–256.

prehospital tools in children yielded poor diagnostic utility and inability to distinguish strokes from mimics in children [303,304]. The adult National Institutes of Health Stroke Scale (NIHSS) score is a validated tool developed for AIS to determine clinical stroke severity based on standard neurological examination findings [305]. The pediatric NIHSS is a modified version of this adult scale, assessing 15 items which have been modified to be developmentally appropriate for children [287,306]. Performing this evaluation remotely can be challenging and comparisons of remote and bedside assessment in the pediatric population are limited.

In order to facilitate making the stroke diagnosis and considering reperfusion therapies, the clinician also needs access to rapid neuroimaging. This poses a challenge in the pediatric population as often in the emergency room, computed tomography—based imaging is more readily available yet is not sensitive for early brain ischemia. Magnetic resonance imaging (MRI) can often definitively differentiate between strokes and mimics but this has some disadvantages. Readily available anesthesiology teams to provide sedation in younger children, longer scan times, and lack of access to MRI after standard business hours can lead to delays in making the diagnosis [299,300].

In 2019, the American Heart Association/American Stroke Association guidelines recommended development of pediatric hyperacute stroke pathways and considering current adult guidelines for arterial recanalization therapy, including intravenous tissue plasminogen activator (tPA) and intraarterial tPA or endovascular thrombectomy [307,308]. These pathways should include criteria for consideration of endovascular thrombectomy in children with acute ischemic stroke and large vessel occlusion. In addition, referral networks should be established to connect community hospitals and frontline providers to tertiary care pediatric stroke centers with specifically trained experts and technology in vascular neurology, neuroimaging, and neurocritical care [309—313]. Telestroke brings expertise to emergency room providers who may have less experience with acute focal deficits and stroke in children [291,292,314,315]. Within pediatric stroke centers, multiple systems of care need to be coordinated through well-designed institutional care protocols which can provide 24/7 access to care from vascular neurologists, vascular neurosurgeons, neuroradiologists, neuro-interventionalists, anesthesiologists, and neurocritical care intensivists [307].

From a clinical standpoint, newborns often present with seizures, typically focal motor seizures involving only one extremity [316,317]. The clinical presentation of acute stroke in children are similar to those in adults. The most common symptoms include hemiparesis and hemifacial weak-ness, speech or language disturbance, vision disturbance, and ataxia. Chil-dren can also present with nonlocalizing symptoms such as headache and altered mental status and seizures at stroke onset are more common in children than adults [286,318,319]. Challenges unique to the telepediatric examination include not being able to reliably assess sensation, reflexes, tone, strength, or fundoscopy via telemedicine [100]. Training courses with interactive pediatric consultations can increase clinicians comfort level with the examination. The advent of apps such as TytoPro and TytoHome for clinician and parent, respectively, provide all in one digital stethoscope, otoscope, thermometer, and camera for streamlined and thorough remote examinations. By using interactive videoconferencing, and the optional use of devices such as stethoscopes, ophthalmoscopes, and ultrasonography machines, patients can simulate an in-person bedside consultation with a pediatric specialist [320]. For pediatric videoconferencing, it is recommended to have an onsite coordinator and distant site coordinator to assist the patient and family to ensure that the technology is functioning properly and to attain vital signs and help with parts of the examination [99].

The pediatric neurological examination can also be limited by technical factors but a young patient may also be reluctant to cooperate particularly in an unfamiliar environment. Although the usual order of the neurological examination may be followed, if some portions cannot be performed properly, such as ophthalmoscopic examination or assessment of tone and deep tendon reflexes, it is important to be flexible and creative with the exam. Additionally, other parts of the neurological examination may be more easily performed by simple observation and detailed testing of gait, balance, and coordination is relatively easy to assess [95,99]. (See Tables 6.2 and 6.3).

The strength of pediatric telestroke lies in its ability to overcome barriers of distance and time to reach medically underserved populations. As technology continues to improve and decrease in cost, telemedicine will improve research, education, access to care, emergency response, and the delivery of specialty pediatrics in diverse settings [135]. As with adult telestroke, the most significant barriers are payment, licensing across state borders, and liability. Pediatric stroke specific guidelines should be developed at the local, regional, and national levels. To leverage regional stroke expertise, partnerships between emergency medical services, comprehensive stroke centers, and pediatric tertiary care hospitals should be encouraged [292,307]. (See Table 6.4).

Table 6.2 Key elements of the pediatric acute telestroke examination (for age 2 and older).

1. Level of consciousness (LOC) (for age 2 and older)
   - Ask the child how old are you (give credit if the child states the correct age or shows the correct number of fingers for his/her age)
   - Ask the child "where is XX?" referring to parent or other familiar person, use the name for that person which the child typically uses (give credit if child correctly points to or gazes purposefully in the direction of the family member)
   - LOC commands: for children one may substitute the command to grip the hand with the command "show me your nose" or "touch your nose"
2. Best gaze:
   - Test horizontal eye movements only, parent or provider can play a game of moving a toy in front of the child's face where patient can only look but not touch. Asking child to look at something also tests joint attention
3. Visual: (upper and lower quadrants)
   - Test by confrontation, using finger counting (for children > 6 years) or visual threat (for children age 2–6 years) as appropriate
4. Facial palsy:
   - Ask, or use pantomime to encourage the patient to show teeth or raise eyebrows and close eyes
5 & 6. Motor arm and leg:
   - The limb is placed in the appropriate position: extend the arms (palms down) 90° (if sitting) or 45° (if supine) and the leg 30° (always tested supine). Drift is scored if the arm falls before 10 s or the leg before 5 s. For children too immature to follow precise directions or uncooperative for any reason, power in each limb should be graded by observation of spontaneous or elicited movement according to the same grading scheme, excluding the time limits
7. Limb ataxia:
   - Test with eyes open. In children, substitute this task with reaching for a toy for the upper extremity, and kicking a toy or the examiner's hand, in children too young (<5 years) or otherwise uncooperative for the standard exam item
8. Sensory:
   - For children too young or otherwise uncooperative for reporting gradations of sensory loss, observe for any behavioral response to pin prick

Continued

Table 6.2 Key elements of the pediatric acute telestroke examination (for age 2 and older).—cont'd

   9. Best language:
- For children age 6 years and up with normal language development before onset of stroke can use PedNIHSS picture, naming and reading sheets
- For children age 2–6 years (or older children with premorbid language skills < 6 yr level), score this item based on observations of language comprehension and speech during the examination

  10. Dysarthria:
- If patient is thought to be normal, an adequate sample of speech must be obtained by asking patient to read or repeat words

  11. Extinction and inattention (formerly neglect):
- Sufficient information to identify neglect may be obtained during the prior testing

Adapted from the Pediatric NIHSS Guide Ichord RN, et al. Interrater reliability of the Pediatric National Institutes of Health Stroke Scale (PedNIHSS) in a multicenter study. Stroke 2011;42(3):613–617 and Child Neurology Society Pediatric Neurological Examination via Telemedicine Grefe A, Hsieh D, Joshi C, Joshi S, Mintz M, Segal M, Shahid A. Pediatric neurological examination via telemedicine 2020.

Table 6.3 Conducting infant and toddler telemedicine examination.

Infant (<12 months):

1. Mental status:
- try to get infant's attention/interaction, or observe the interaction of the infant with the caregiver—smile, funny faces, play "peek-a-boo."

2. Visual fields:
- have caregiver hold a toy 1–2 feet in front of child's face with one hand; with the other hand slowly approach child's peripheral vision from behind and watch for child shifting attention to the new object.

3. Facial palsy:
- easy to assess visually, ideally in neutral affect and while smiling/laughing/crying.

4. Motor:
- start with observation, are movements normal and symmetric? Have caregiver gently pull on each limb and release—normal recoil response?
- if child is able to creep/crawl, observe him/her doing so—if the child is already able to stand/cruise, observe cruising and have child walk from one caregiver to the other with one- or two-hand assist. Focus camera on lower extremities.
- have caregiver offer a toy to the child in midline—make sure camera angle is such that you can observe for premature hand preference and overt tremor/dysmetria. Once child has the toy in his/her grasp, have caregiver try to playfully take the toy away and have them report on any obvious asymmetry.

(Continued)

Table 6.3 Conducting infant and toddler telemedicine examination.—cont'd

5. Sensory
- with child in caregiver's lap or on a flat surface, have the child focus on a visually interesting toy or noise maker and gently tickle different parts of the body, judging reaction.

Toddler (12–36 months):

Similar to infant testing.
- If toddler appears to be developmentally normal will also follow commands to look toward mommy/daddy (right/left), "show me all your teeth," "roar like a lion" (open mouth).
- to test motor strength, have toddlers do the chicken dance (tests deltoids by inspection)/sing "head- shoulders-knees-and-toes" while touching body parts—tests strength as well as coordination.

Adapted from the Pediatric NIHSS Guide Ichord RN, et al. Interrater reliability of the Pediatric National Institutes of Health Stroke Scale (PedNIHSS) in a multicenter study. Stroke 2011;42(3):613–617 and Child Neurology Society Pediatric Neurological Examination via Telemedicine Grefe A, Hsieh D, Joshi C, Joshi S, Mintz M, Segal M, Shahid A. Pediatric neurological examination via telemedicine, 2020.

Table 6.4 Pediatric telestroke barriers and benefits of implementation.

Aspects of care	Benefits	Barriers
Access to care	• Timely access to specialist • Reduces disparities • Strengthens relationship between ED providers and stroke experts	• Changes the traditional patient—doctor relationship • Technical knowledge • Language barriers
Evaluation	• May improve timeliness to diagnosis and treatment • Standardized workflows	• Difficulty in performing the remote examination • Difficulty in obtaining neuroimaging
Education	• Improves stroke awareness • Continuing medical education • Facilitates patient selection in clinical trials	• Language barriers • Need to train staff at originating site
Resource utilization	• Potential to shorten hospital stay • May avoid unnecessary transfers • Leadership support • Quality improvement efforts	• Limited studies on reliability, validity, safety, efficacy, and cost-effectiveness • Systematic data collection • Liability, confidentiality, and regulatory concerns

Modified from Uscher-Pines L, Kahn JM. Barriers and facilitators to pediatric emergency telemedicine in the United States. Telemed J Health 2014;20(11):990–996.

CHAPTER 7

Barriers, legal issues, and limitations

Telemedicine is increasingly seen as a key component of healthcare in the future. The expansion of telestroke has led to more efficient and affordable stroke care. This expansion decreases barriers associated with distance, cost, provider and patient time, and limit use of stretched resources in the emergency department. However, there are several barriers to overcome in order to implement telestroke into routine clinical practice. Challenges such as technical, administrative, and operational infrastructure can make growth of a telestroke practice difficult. However, none were more challenging than the COVID-19 pandemic which propelled the growth of telemedicine and acceptance of telemedicine. While the pandemic led to changes and relaxation of certain rules, it is not clear that these will prevail long term. Determining reimbursement models that can support a practice, credential providers, improve interfaces, obtain less-costly equipment, and most importantly develop evidence-based standards for care is a priority for global acceptance of telestroke [134].

Professional licensure and credentialing

In the United States, the responsibility for licensing and otherwise regulating health professionals lies with state governments. All states require physicians, nurses, dentists, and certain other healthcare personnel to be licensed by the state to practice their profession. The penalties for practicing medicine without a license are significant and may include criminal as well as civil penalties. Barriers to telestroke implementation in the United States include the lack of nationwide credentialing and licensing. Telemedicine can complicate decisions about where a practitioner should be licensed if the practitioner and patient are located in different states. Credentialing often involves completion of arduous and

TeleStroke
ISBN 978-0-12-824161-5
https://doi.org/10.1016/B978-0-12-824161-5.00007-4

© 2021 Elsevier Inc.
All rights reserved.

redundant paperwork for each spoke site. The Centers for Medicare & Medicaid Services' (CMS's) Final Rule published in May 5, 2011, amended the conditions of participation with respect to the requirements for credentialing and privileging related to telemedicine services. This regulation, allows for "credentialing by proxy," permitting spoke hospitals to rely on the credentialing and privileging decisions of the hub hospital [95,135]. However, many community hospitals refuse to do so out of fear of liability concerns, professional staff bylaw restrictions, and certain states have opted not to allow credentialing by proxy [136]. Some states are making it easier for physicians to practice in other states. The Interstate Medical Licensure Compact encompasses 28 states and the territory of Guam and their 38 medical and osteopathic boards and offers an "expedited pathway to licensure for qualified physicians" seeking to practice in multiple states. It also offers reciprocity, with the members recognizing each other's licensing requirements [125].

Some telemedicine programs are not affected as they operate entirely within a single state. Programs operated by the federal government are not restricted by state licensure laws and healthcare providers working in the military, the Department of Veterans Affairs, the US Public Health Service, and the federal prison system can proceed with cross-state tests and applications of telemedicine without concern about state challenges or penalties. Availability of a national or multistate license would reduce the need for a consultant to be licensed in multiple states and reduce the significant administrative burden on clinicians and telestroke networks [126].

Personal barriers

Telemedicine challenges the traditional view of professional practice as involving a face-to-face encounter between clinician and patient. There is a concern that this platform is impersonal and leads to disruption of the doctor–patient relationship [95,137]. Personal barriers to telestroke are usually related to provider acceptance, patient acceptance, and personnel training. Concerns regarding inadequate training and technical problems, ease of use, imaging resolution, and perceived usefulness must be allayed in order to gain acceptance. Glitches or sound/video delays can impede the flow of normal conversation. Providers tend to be the most cautious in accepting telestroke [138]. Telestroke evaluations are not easily integrated into routine workflow, adds extra time to already busy schedules, and can be perceived as adding little benefit beyond a traditional telephone call [139]. Consultant physicians also do not want to be perceived as "stepping on the toes" of community physicians. Community providers perceive the consultant as a supervisor and are distrustful of consultants they do not know [140,141]. Patients may have an inadequate perception of the telemedicine and hesitant to use it. Studies have demonstrated positive improvement in their acceptance and understanding after experiencing the service [142,143].

Also, remote visits require patients to have the knowledge and capacity to get online, operate and trouble shoot audiovisual equipment. Older adults account for 25% of physician office visits in the United States and often have multiple morbidities and disabilities. Thirteen million older adults may have trouble accessing telemedical services; a disproportionate number of those may be among the already disadvantaged. Older adults may be unable to do this as a result of inexperience with technologies or disabilities [144,145]. Telephone visits may improve access for the estimated 6.3 million older adults who are inexperienced with technology or have visual impairment, but phone visits are suboptimal for care that requires visual assessment [146–148].

Legal issues

Legal parameters must be established to facilitate the use of telestroke. A significant issue concerns medicolegal liability. Clear liability protections must be in place at both sites to protect the consulting providers and the providers following the remote consultant's advice [135]. In order to write a prescription in the United States, a clinician must have a license to practice in the state where the patient is located. Transmission of the consultation occurs via the public Internet, ensuring appropriate encryption to satisfy HIPAA requirements and ensure patient data safety and confidentiality is also important [140,149]. Research on telephone malpractice cases has found them to be extremely costly with regard to settlements, and results in significant morbidity and even mortality [150]. According to multistate legal claims, providers have the potential to be open to suits in two locations: the state where the hub is located and the state where the spoke is located [151]. Overall, physicians who comply with licensing rules, who document appropriately and who follow the same standards of care they would for in-person treatments may not have additional malpractice risks for a virtual visit. Consultation with legal team and malpractice insurance company prior to starting telemedicine services is recommended. It is also unclear what might happen in the case of technology failure in the hyperacute stroke decision-making process. States also require physicians to obtain consent from patients before treating them, but some states have specific requirements around consent that others do not. California, for instance, requires the originating site provider to obtain and document patient consent, according to the Center for Connected Health Policy, while Kentucky says the treating physician who delivers or facilitates the telemedicine services is responsible for obtaining consent [124]. The risk of legal action can be mitigated by careful documentation of the telestroke consultation and periodic quality review of consultations by peer review. Understanding informed refusal is also important. While a practice should work to accommodate the preferences of a patient, patients need to understand that there are conditions and circumstances where an in-person visit may be necessary. Documenting refusal of care is important, especially when the physician feels the patient warrants an in-person evaluation but the patient refuses to do so even when the potential risks were explained. Consider using a Refusal of Care form, if signed by the physician with a staff member as a witness this can mitigate liability [152].

Cost/reimbursement

The development of telemedicine programs for the treatment of stroke requires capital investment in infrastructure. Practices must invest large upfront costs for equipment and startup and have continued costs of equipment maintenance, personnel training, and ongoing technical support. For rural and underserved areas, this is particularly challenging in maintaining sustainability [153]. The capital investment for a telemedicine program is estimated to ranging from $46,000 up to a high cost of $200,000 or more per spoke [154]. Decision-analytic models show that telestroke is cost-effective from both a societal and a hospital perspective [155]. To evaluate the cost-effectiveness of telestroke services, researchers at the University of Utah Stroke Center developed a decision-analytic model that used the cost of treatment with the use of telestroke consultation and the quality of life after treatment for both 90-day and lifetime horizons. The costs and benefits were compared with the costs and quality of life of patients treated in rural emergency rooms without the assistance of a neurologist via telemedicine. The study concluded that telestroke may be cost-effective in the long term, but during the short term, it does not seem to be cost-effective because of large upfront fixed equipment costs. Systematic reviews have found no evidence that telehealth interventions are cost-effective compared with conventional healthcare [155]. Telestroke programs often look to government or foundations to help with these significant upfront capital expenses but this is often not sufficient for long-term sustainability.

Reimbursement is a significant barrier to widespread acceptance of telestroke. There is a lack of clear and consistent reimbursement and return on investment. Medical necessity for telemedicine services must satisfy the requirements for concurrent care services. Concurrent care exists when >1 provider is required to address the clinical needs of a patient [156,157]. Typically, this situation arises when the opinion of another provider with specific clinical expertise is required to treat a presenting problem such as rendering a diagnosis or developing a treatment plan. Medicare reimbursement is difficult and requires certain service locations and sites in order to receive payment. There is no universal reimbursement policy for telehealth encounters, and many insurers only reimburse for in-person service. As of 2007, a total of 35 states allowed for some reimbursement services, although not all states required reimbursement at the same rate as in-person encounters.

In 2010, the Center for Medicare and Medicaid Services established a consultation code for telehealth; however, its use is limited to hospitals outside of metropolitan areas [139]. The codes are time based and not recognized by most non-Medicare payers. Many payers recognize CPT-4 codes approved for telemedicine, such as evaluation and management services (CPT codes 99201 through 99233). However, these codes do not adequately describe the service provided. Furthermore, some of these services require the documentation and performance of a comprehensive physical examination, which is not practical for a provider in a distant hospital [157]. As a result of the time consuming process for reimbursement, many programs fail to complete billing adequately even when a payor may reimburse [135,139]. Reimbursement for telestroke services should not be based on a facility's rural or urban location but should be applicable anywhere the services are available.

Current Procedural Terminology (CPT) codes need to be updated to include services such as telestroke and should include specific codes for the patient monitoring and management that is needed in a remote facility. Further research using a systematic review with a meta-analysis should be performed to provide a more precise measurement of the effects (e.g., costs, savings, and reimbursement) of the implementation and maintenance of telestroke programs in healthcare facilities using technology [154]. Misaligned incentives have also been reported as a barrier in studies of telehealth where it may benefit the individual patient (such as getting to stay in a community hospital while avoiding transport to an academic medical center far from home) but no benefit or sometimes a disincentive, for the physicians involved [139,155].

Several states, including California and Georgia, have recently updated their laws to improve access to telehealth services. These laws establish payment parity for telehealth services allowing providers to be reimbursed at the same rate as they would for in-person services. Several states are also establishing laws regarding remote patient monitoring and store-and-forward services. This will greatly help elderly patients, patients with chronic conditions, or postsurgical patients who may be too ill or not have the necessary resources to obtain an in-person visit.

Technology and connectivity

"Information technology must play a central role in the redesign of the health care system if a substantial improvement in quality is to be achieved" [24]. Spoke facilities use a variety of technologies to support a telestroke network. Silva et al. reported that in 56% of hubs, the systems used could interact only with other systems of the same model by the same manufacturer [158]. In addition, rural spoke sites may need to build interfaces for data storage and retrieval with an electronic health record system adding cost as well as experienced IT needs [158]. Initial videoconferencing technology required the remote neurologist to be present at a fixed workstation but technical advances have since led to laptop- and smartphone-based videoconferencing [29,159,160]. Telestroke networks need to be HIPAA compliant as they can be vulnerable due to multiple areas in which data breaches can occur. Data security with end-to-end, reliable documentation and storage and strict control of access to users within the network is vital but can be expensive for a telestroke practice. Cyber liability assessment ensures the practice has the proper security controls in place as any device connected to the network can provide an entry point to a practice. The practice should review insurance coverage to ensure protection from cybersecurity attack. Cyber risk is of significant concern. Although some states have relaxed restrictions around non-HIPAA compliant platforms, try to utilize a compliant one. "Zoom-bombing" during a consultation and other scenarios in which hackers can cause a breach leading to patient privacy issues can lead to disruption in the network or practice. This can lead to business interruption, lawsuits, and fines. If a practice is upgrading or purchasing new technology, it is important to adjust security settings and turn on controls to ensure privacy protection [161].

CHAPTER 8

Novel technologies and clinical applications

The evolution of medical technology over the decades has propelled clinical care into an era of faster, more flexible, and accessible care. The benefits to patients, families, caregivers, and treatment teams are significant. However, this relationship needs to work seamlessly in the structural environments of clinical care and performing randomized clinical trials to assess benefit with the rapidly changing technology is not an easy endeavor. Several innovative technologies that have had an impact on clinical care include telepresence, virtual reality (VR), augmented reality (AR), and remote monitoring systems [192]. The definitions are refined, combined, and classified in different ways and often used interchangeably which can sometimes be challenging. However, these novel technologies have potential to impact care of patients in many ways.

Telepresence (TPr) refers to the use of VR technology, especially for remote control of machinery or for apparent participation in distant events. VR is defined as an artificial environment which is experienced through multisensory stimuli (such as sights and sounds) provided by a computer and in which one's actions partially determine what happens in the environment. AR is an enhanced version of reality created by the use of technology to overlay digital information on an image of something being viewed through a device (such as a smartphone camera). Mixed reality is considered a combination of VR and AR. Remote patient monitoring (RPM) uses digital technologies to collect medical and other forms of health data from individuals in one location and electronically transmit that information securely to healthcare providers in a different location for assessment and recommendations [193] (See Fig. 8.1).

VR/AR technology have been used for cardiac rehabilitation, medicine, pain management, surgical procedures palliative care, and neurological disorders [194–199]. VR technology is also used as adjunctive therapy in neuro-rehabilitation where it has potential regarding repetition, intensity, and task-oriented training of a paretic extremity [200–202]. VR can also be used in patients with Parkinson's disease where AR feedback on performance enables repetitive practice of motor tasks and stimulates motor and

TeleStroke
ISBN 978-0-12-824161-5
https://doi.org/10.1016/B978-0-12-824161-5.00008-6

© 2021 Elsevier Inc.
All rights reserved.

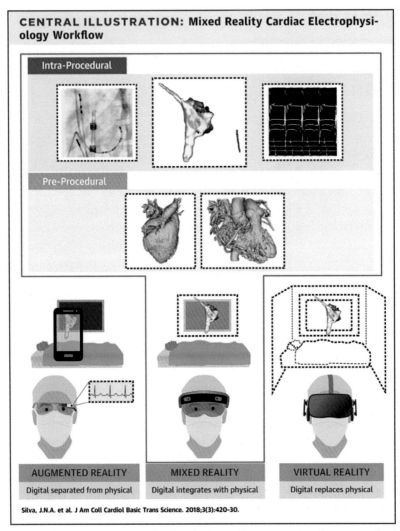

Figure 8.1 Mixed reality allows for the display and interaction with existing displays within the cardiac catheterization suite, including integration with fluoroscopy **(top left)**, electroanatomic mapping systems **(top center)**, electrocardiograms **(top right)**, as well as previously acquired and computed tomography- or magnetic resonance–derived three-dimensional (3D) anatomic models **(middle row)**. Although augmented reality platforms **(bottom left)** can show two-dimensional (2D) data unobtrusively, mixed reality platforms **(bottom center)** allow for hands-free 2D and 3D visualization as well as direct sterile control of these data without otherwise obstructing the normal visual field, as in virtual reality **(bottom right)** [192].

cognitive processes simultaneously [203]. VR allows users to interact with a multisensory environment and receive "real-time" feedback on performance in a nonimmersive to fully immersive virtual environment. This depends on the degree to which the user is isolated from the physical surroundings during the interaction [204−209]. Nonimmersive commercial video game systems (e.g., Wii, Kinect, PlayStation) are also classified as VR and as they are more readily available and less costly can be adapted for clinical use [209]. In a metaanalysis of VR in stroke rehabilitation, researchers reported that VR and video game applications are potentially useful technologies that can be combined with conventional rehabilitation for upper arm improvement after stroke [207]. Home-based telerehabilitation, where a healthcare professional oversees the rehabilitation process from a remote location, has been shown to be a valuable and feasible alternative for patients with limited access to traditional rehabilitation [38]. Telerehabilitation has been reported to improve the health of patients poststroke, including upper extremity function, while also being supportive of caregiver's needs [210,211].

Several new devices to help identify large vessel occlusions in the field are presently in development. The volumetric impedance phase shift spectroscopy (VIPS) device (Cerebrotech, Pleasanton, California) has demonstrated high sensitivity and specificity in detecting large vessel occlusions in stroke patients [212]. The VIPS device can detect regions of ischemia, which correlate to an LVO. The SONAS device (BURL Concepts, San Diego, California) uses transcranial ultrasound and microbubble intravenous contrast to identify potential LVOs [188]. This technology can be deployed in the field in an attempt to expedite diagnosis and triage to an appropriate medical center. Clinical trials are ongoing.

Artificial intelligence (AI) aims to mimic human cognitive functions. AI and machine learning software are being used more commonly for diagnostic purposes [213]. Increasing access to healthcare data and analytical techniques created a paradigm change in stroke management [213]. These algorithms are self-learning and can enhance and expedite been used stroke diagnostic recognition [188]. Viz LVO (Viz.ai, San Francisco, California) uses an algorithm to detect suspected LVOs on CT angiography and subsequently alerts stroke specialists in minutes [214,215]. Both an alert and postprocessed images are sent to the mobile devices of members of an assigned stroke team, including radiologists, neurologists, and neurointerventionalists. The application contains a HIPAA compliant messaging service and recently obtained de novo FDA clearance for clinical use. This is the first time CMS has reimbursed an AI-based software using this designation [214,215].

Telerobotic stroke intervention may provide a novel solution for interventional stroke management at smaller regional or rural healthcare systems. These telerobotic devices are capable of conducting endovascular thrombectomy and have been studied both in vitro and in vivo models [216–218]. However, there are several challenges with telerobotic care such as operational and financial considerations. Corindus Vascular Robotics developed the CorPAth GRX device for percutaneous coronary intervention (PCI) as demonstrated in the PRECISE (Percutaneous Robotically-Enhanced Coronary Intervention) and CORA-PCI (Complex Robotically Assisted Percutaneous Coronary Intervention) trials [216,219,220]. Studies have demonstrated that the device is adaptable to neuroendovascular procedures such as transradial carotid artery stenting [221]. The system allows a physician to sit at a remote radiation–shielded workstation and use a set of touchscreen controls and joysticks that are then translated to the movements of the local robotic device. The robotic unit includes all the usual endovascular tools such as angiographic and hemodynamic monitors, foot pedal controlled fluoroscopy [221]. Further research and development of neuroendovascular robotics is needed (see Fig. 8.2).

RPM systems provide another novel approach to stroke patients. Wearable, wireless motion sensors can analyze mobility-related activities using activity pattern-recognition algorithms to describe the type, quantity, and quality of patient activities which can guide treatment [222,223]. Data transmission from sensors to a cell phone and Internet enable continuous monitoring and remote access to data about walking speed, duration and distance, gait asymmetry and smoothness of movements, as well as cycling, exercise, and skills practice, offers unique opportunities to engage patients in progressive, personalized therapies with feedback about performance [222,223].

RPM devices (connected health devices) include wearable heart monitors, bluetooth-enabled scales, Fitbits and smart watches, blood pressure telemonitoring, glucometers from an increasing number of RPM vendors [224]. These RPM technologies automatically observe and report on patients, often with chronic illnesses, so healthcare providers can remotely facilitate healthcare decisions. Not only do these devices empower patients to better manage their health and participate in their healthcare but they also provide a comprehensive view of a patient's health over time, increase visibility into a patient's adherence to a treatment, and enable timely intervention before a costly care episode

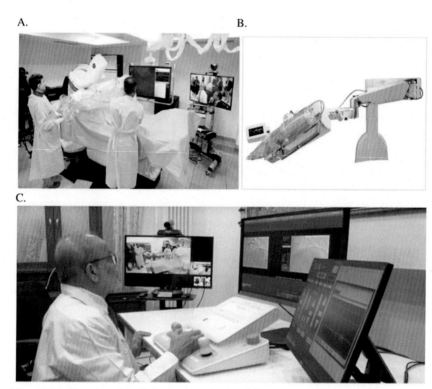

Figure 8.2 Photographs of the catheterization laboratory (A), CorPath GRX bedside Robotic Arm (B), Cassette and Remote Robotic Control Work Station (C) [257].

[101,225,226]. Clinicians can strengthen their relationships with their patients by using the data sent to them via RPM to develop a personalized care plan and to engage in joint decision-making to foster better outcomes [101,225,226]. Apple is testing whether its Apple Watch can be used to detect irregular heart patterns, and AliveCor's KardiaBand allows Apple Watch wearers to perform electrocardiograms in 30 s that can easily be transmitted to physicians [227,228]. Other new-at-home devices can allow patients to complete an ultrasound using a phone app or screen for hypertension while at a barbershop.

The integration of mobile communications with wearable sensors has facilitated the shift to patient-centric delivery models and hopefully will impact the clinical and economic burden of chronic disease management. The positive effects of RPM have been reported in cardiovascular and cerebrovascular disease such as hypertension, heart failure, and atrial fibrillation [229–234]. During the COVID-19 pandemic, connected health and RPM are valuable tools as patients can be monitored closely without contact, allowing them to be managed remotely preserving bed space for critically ill patients [235]. Barriers to this technology include integration of the data into healthcare systems while protecting patient safety, understanding the end-users' needs to inform system design, randomized controlled trials to conclusively demonstrate benefit of use (reduced hospitalization rates, reduction in mortality compared to traditional in person follow-up and the degree of impact of RPM) [236–238].

Virtual telestroke support is commonly used in the Emergency Department using various telehealth solutions. Hands-free wearable technology can also combine AR/VR platforms to allow for seamless communication, improved real-time capabilities, and faster more informed decisions. It can advance the triage of stroke patients into the prehospital setting at the scene or in the ambulance and facilitate the routing of patients to comprehensive stroke centers. Devices such as Xpert Eye solution, a Google Glass-based wearable solution, and Vuzix telemedicine Smart Glasses are uniquely helpful where onsite care practitioner can receive live expert interactive medical feedback while simultaneously acting on the feedback in evaluating patients with suspected acute stroke [239]. Telemedicine via smart glasses is being used for virtual ICU rounds in neurosurgical patients and reported to be feasible, effective, and widely accepted as an alternative to physical ward rounds during the COVID-19 pandemic [240]. These devices also have application in the ambulatory and home setting where nurses and other healthcare practitioners can perform wound care and medication checks in person with real-time feedback and consultation with a remote provider [241]. Barriers include poor camera image preventing from wider use in telemedicine, short battery life, memory limits, wearability and patient confidentiality, and sensitive data storage and transmission (Fig. 8.3).

TPr robots can augment the clinician/patient interaction by adding a human-sized physical embodiment and enhanced control for the remote user [242]. Systems include screen-based TPr robots to android representations of the remote provider. The remote provider uses a camera, mobile base, and mannerisms to augment video or audio communication to the local person with the system [193,242]. Surgical robotic integrative technology such as the da Vinci telerobotic system has improved procedures, reduced cost and recovery times [243–245]. Robotic TPr can also improve communication between people with dementia, family, and staff and enables customized care [246–250]. Several telestroke networks have

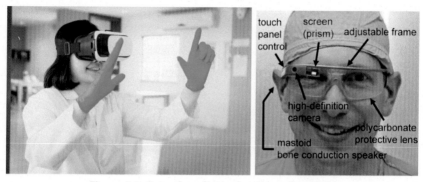

Figure 8.3 Examples of virtual reality technology.

successfully implemented the use of TPr robots for both emergency stroke and inpatient access to stroke experts. Use of the TPr technology has shown improved physician rapid response to unstable ICU patients and the stroke expert uses a laptop and wireless Internet to connect to the TPr robot in community and rural hospitals, improving patient outcomes, decreased length of ICU stay, decreased cost, and immediate access to stroke and neurocritical care specialists [98,251—256]. Barriers include large upfront costs for equipment, staff training, sufficient connection bandwidth, adequate access to electronic health records, and data integration.

CHAPTER 9

The future of telestroke

Although telestroke was part of the delivery of care in the United States for many years, its use accelerated rapidly when the COVID-19 pandemic struck in January 2020. Telestroke has shifted the paradigm of acute stroke treatment by supporting hospitals without stroke care expertise to improve patient access to recommended treatments. A recent study found that approximately a quarter of hospitals now have access to this technology for patients in their emergency departments [329]. While telestroke has bridged some of the gaps in geographic disparities in stroke care, it still appears that smaller, rural, and critical access hospitals, the group of hospitals that might benefit most from telestroke are relatively less likely to have adopted this technology [329]. Telestroke certainly has the potential to reduce healthcare costs, improve health outcomes, and increase patient outreach. As the technology advances, more widespread adoption may help close the gaps in stroke care and tackle disparities which arise due to proximity to healthcare providers. As telestroke accelerates its reach more broadly, it will increase operational efficiencies and allow clinicians to treat patients and manage stroke patients anywhere.

Many of the prepandemic barriers to more widespread adoption of telestroke such as lack of capital investment, reimbursement, privacy, and regulatory barriers have only been temporarily relaxed. Unless Congress acts, these barriers will return after the public health emergency is over. We need to optimize long-term telehealth policies and create regulatory changes to efficiently and successfully incorporate telehealth into our new standard of care post pandemic. We need to accelerate telehealth development, quantify clinical outcomes, and build on the current telestroke structure. A unified effort will help increase telestroke adoption rates and allow for exponential growth of telestroke programs, further expanding a new era in healthcare delivery.

TeleStroke
ISBN 978-0-12-824161-5
https://doi.org/10.1016/B978-0-12-824161-5.00009-8

© 2021 Elsevier Inc.
All rights reserved.

References

[1] WHO Group Consultation on Health Telematics (1997: Geneva Switzerland), Lederberg J, World Health Organization. A health telematics policy in support of WHO's Health-For-All Strategy for Global Development : report of the WHO Group Consultation on Health Telematics, 11–16 December, Geneva, 1997. Geneva: World Health Organization; 1998. p. 39.

[2] Ryu S. History of telemedicine: evolution, context, and transformation. Healthcare Inf Res 2010;16(1):65–6.

[3] Bashshur R, National Library of Medicine (U.S.). The history of telemedicine. Bethesda, MD: National Library of Medicine; 2009.

[4] Bashshur R, Shannon GW. History of telemedicine: evolution, context, and transformation. New Rochelle, NY: Mary Ann Liebert; 2009. p. 415.

[5] Nesbitt T. The evolution of telehealth: where have we been and where are we going?. In: The role of telehealth in an evolving health care environment: workshop summary. Washington, DC: The National Academic Press; 2012. p. 11–5.

[6] Einthoven W. The telecardiogram. Am Heart J 1957;53(4):602–15.

[7] The radio doctor - maybe! Radio News Mag 1924.

[8] Zundel KM. Telemedicine: history, applications, and impact on librarianship. Bull Med Libr Assoc 1996;84(1):71–9.

[9] Gershon-Cohen J, Cooley AG. Telognosis. Radiology 1950;55(4):582–7.

[10] Allen A. From early wireless to Everest. Telemed Today 1998;6(2):16–8.

[11] Allen A. Cutting edge Internet teleradiology from nine leading vendors. Telemed Today 1998;6(3):15–7.

[12] Wachter G, Brown N, Allen A. Teleradiology service providers. Telemed Today 1996;4(6):14–5. 30.

[13] Benschoter RA, Television V. Multi-purpose television. Ann NY Acad Sci 1967;142(2):471–8.

[14] Benschoter RA, Eaton MT, Smith P. Use of videotape to provide individual instruction in techniques of psychotherapy. J Med Educ 1965;40(12):1159–61.

[15] Benschoter RA, Nelle J, Karlins M. Producing mental health teaching materials. Hosp Community Psychiatry 1967;18(4):122–4.

[16] Benschoter RA, Wittson CL, Ingham CG. Teaching and consultation by television. I. Closed-circuit collaboration. Ment Hosp 1965;16:99–100.

[17] Cermack M. Monitoring and telemedicine support in remote environments and in human space flight. Br J Anaesth 2006;97(1):107–14.

[18] Perednia DA. Telemedicine system evaluation and a collaborative model for multi-centered research. J Med Syst 1995;19(3):287–94.

[19] Perednia DA, Allen A. Telemedicine technology and clinical applications. JAMA 1995;273(6):483–8.

[20] Perednia DA, Brown NA. Teledermatology: one application of telemedicine. Bull Med Libr Assoc 1995;83(1):42–7.

[21] Perednia DA, Gaines JA, Butruille TW. Comparison of the clinical informativeness of photographs and digital imaging media with multiple-choice receiver operating characteristic analysis. Arch Dermatol 1995;131(3):292–7.

[22] Scannell K, et al., Telemedicine: past, present, future: January 1966 through March 1995: 1634 citations. Current bibliographies in medicine. 1995, Bethesda, MD. (8600 Rockville Pike) Pittsburgh, PA: U.S. Dept. of Health and Human Services, Public

Health Service, National Institutes of Health, National Library of Medicine Sold by the Supt. of Docs., U.S. G.P.O. ix, pp. 123.

[23] Crump WJ, Pfeil T. A telemedicine primer. An introduction to the technology and an overview of the literature. Arch Fam Med 1995;4(9):796—803. Discussion 804.

[24] Field MJ, editor. Telemedicine: a guide to assessing telecommunications in health care; 1996. Washington (DC).

[25] United States. Congress. Office of Technology Assessment., Health care in rural America. Washington, DC: Congress of the U.S., Office of Technology Assessment : For sale by the Supt. of Docs., U.S. G.P.O; 1990. p. 529.

[26] Levine SR, Gorman M. "Telestroke": the application of telemedicine for stroke. Stroke 1999;30(2):464—9.

[27] Schwamm LH, et al. Virtual TeleStroke support for the emergency department evaluation of acute stroke. Acad Emerg Med 2004;11(11):1193—7.

[28] LaMonte MP, et al. Telemedicine for acute stroke: triumphs and pitfalls. Stroke 2003;34(3):725—8.

[29] Shafqat S, et al. Role for telemedicine in acute stroke. Feasibility and reliability of remote administration of the NIH stroke scale. Stroke 1999;30(10):2141—5.

[30] Akbik F, et al. Telestroke-the promise and the challenge. Part one: growth and current practice. J Neurointerv Surg 2017;9(4):357—60.

[31] Akbik F, et al. Telestroke-the promise and the challenge. Part two-expansion and horizons. J Neurointerv Surg 2017;9(4):361—5.

[32] Moskowitz A, et al. Emergency physician and stroke specialist beliefs and expectations regarding telestroke. Stroke 2010;41(4):805—9.

[33] Benjamin EJ, et al. Heart disease and stroke statistics-2019 update: A report from the American Heart Association. Circulation 2019;139(10):e56—528.

[34] Taylor TN. The medical economics of stroke. Drugs 1997;54(Suppl 3):51—7. Discussion 57-8.

[35] Taylor TN, et al. Lifetime cost of stroke in the United States. Stroke 1996;27(9):1459—66.

[36] Jozefowicz RF. Neurology residency training in the US and Poland. Nat Clin Pract Neurol 2007;3(10):586—7.

[37] Adornato BT, et al. The practice of neurology, 2000—2010: report of the AAN member research subcommittee. Neurology 2011;77(21):1921—8.

[38] Schwamm LH, et al. Recommendations for the implementation of telemedicine within stroke systems of care: a policy statement from the American Heart Association. Stroke 2009;40(7):2635—60.

[39] Schwamm LH, et al. A review of the evidence for the use of telemedicine within stroke systems of care: a scientific statement from the American Heart Association/ American Stroke Association. Stroke 2009;40(7):2616—34.

[40] Freeman WD, et al. Neurohospitalists reduce length of stay for patients with ischemic stroke. Neurohospitalist 2011;1(2):67—70.

[41] Josephson SA, Douglas VC. Neurohospitalist: a newly popular career choice. Neurol Clin Pract 2011;1(1):55—60.

[42] Cronin CA, Weisman CJ, Llinas RH. Stroke treatment: beyond the three-hour window and in the pregnant patient. Ann NY Acad Sci 2008;1142:159—78.

[43] Del Zoppo GJ, et al. Expansion of the time window for treatment of acute ischemic stroke with intravenous tissue plasminogen activator: a science advisory from the American Heart Association/American Stroke Association. Stroke 2009;40(8):2945—8.

[44] Hacke W, et al. Thrombolysis with alteplase 3 to 4.5 hours after acute ischemic stroke. N Engl J Med 2008;359(13):1317—29.

[45] Fagan SC, et al. Cost-effectiveness of tissue plasminogen activator for acute ischemic stroke. NINDS rt-PA Stroke Study Group. Neurology 1998;50(4):883—90.

[46] Lattimore SU, et al. Impact of establishing a primary stroke center at a community hospital on the use of thrombolytic therapy: the NINDS Suburban Hospital Stroke Center experience. Stroke 2003;34(6):e55—7.

[47] Adeoye O, et al. Recombinant tissue-type plasminogen activator use for ischemic stroke in the United States: a doubling of treatment rates over the course of 5 years. Stroke 2011;42(7):1952—5.

[48] Kleindorfer D, et al. US geographic distribution of rt-PA utilization by hospital for acute ischemic stroke. Stroke 2009;40(11):3580—4.

[49] Tong D, et al. Times from symptom onset to hospital arrival in the get with the guidelines–Stroke program 2002 to 2009: temporal trends and implications. Stroke 2012;43(7):1912—7.

[50] Freeman WD, et al. The Workforce Task Force report: clinical implications for neurology. Neurology 2013;81(5):479—86.

[51] Bobrow BJ, et al. Views of emergency physicians on thrombolysis for acute ischemic stroke. J Brain Dis 2009;1:29—37.

[52] Brown DL, et al. Survey of emergency physicians about recombinant tissue plasminogen activator for acute ischemic stroke. Ann Emerg Med 2005;46(1):56—60.

[53] Miley ML, et al. The state of emergency stroke resources and care in rural Arizona: a platform for telemedicine. Telemed J E Health 2009;15(7):691—9.

[54] Demaerschalk BM, et al. Stroke telemedicine. Mayo Clin Proc 2009;84(1):53—64.

[55] Wechsler LR, et al. Telemedicine quality and outcomes in stroke: a scientific statement for healthcare professionals from the American Heart Association/American Stroke Association. Stroke 2017;48(1):e3—25.

[56] Pervez MA, et al. Remote supervision of IV-tPA for acute ischemic stroke by telemedicine or telephone before transfer to a regional stroke center is feasible and safe. Stroke 2010;41(1):e18—24.

[57] Cutting S, et al. Telestroke in an urban setting. Telemed J E Health 2014;20(9):855—7.

[58] Meyer BC, et al. Prospective reliability of the STRokE DOC wireless/site independent telemedicine system. Neurology 2005;64(6):1058—60.

[59] Amorim E, et al. Impact of telemedicine implementation in thrombolytic use for acute ischemic stroke: the University of Pittsburgh Medical Center telestroke network experience. J Stroke Cerebrovasc Dis 2013;22(4):527—31.

[60] Wang S, et al. Remote evaluation of acute ischemic stroke: reliability of National Institutes of Health Stroke Scale via telestroke. Stroke 2003;34(10):e188—91.

[61] Demaerschalk BM, Kiernan TE, Investigators S. Vascular neurology nurse practitioner provision of telemedicine consultations. Int J Telemed Appl 2010;2010.

[62] Meyer BC, et al. Reliability of site-independent telemedicine when assessed by telemedicine-naive stroke practitioners. J Stroke Cerebrovasc Dis 2008;17(4):181—6.

[63] Audebert HJ, et al. Can telemedicine contribute to fulfill WHO Helsingborg Declaration of specialized stroke care? Cerebrovasc Dis 2005;20(5):362—9.

[64] Audebert HJ, et al. Telemedicine stroke department network. Introduction of a telemedicine pilot project for integrated stroke management in South Bavaria and analysis of its efficiency. Nervenarzt 2004;75(2):161—5.

[65] Wiborg A, Widder B, Telemedicine in Stroke in Swabia P. Teleneurology to improve stroke care in rural areas: the Telemedicine in Stroke in Swabia (TESS) Project. Stroke 2003;34(12):2951—6.

[66] Powers WJ, et al. Guidelines for the early management of patients with acute ischemic stroke: 2019 update to the 2018 guidelines for the early management of acute ischemic stroke: a guideline for healthcare professionals from the American Heart Association/American Stroke Association. Stroke 2019;50(12):e344—418.

[67] Solenski NJ. Telestroke. Neuroimaging Clin N Am 2018;28(4):551—63.

[68] Schwamm L, Kaste M, Lee T. Successful networks in resource rich and poor, urban and rural regions. Int J Stroke 2019.

[69] Walter S, et al. Diagnosis and treatment of patients with stroke in a mobile stroke unit versus in hospital: a randomised controlled trial. Lancet Neurol 2012;11(5):397—404.

[70] Ebinger M, et al. Effects of golden hour thrombolysis: a prehospital acute neurological treatment and optimization of medical care in stroke (PHANTOM-S) substudy. JAMA Neurol 2015;72(1):25—30.

[71] Ebinger M, et al. Association between dispatch of mobile stroke units and functional outcomes among patients with acute ischemic stroke in Berlin. JAMA 2021;325(5):454—66.

[72] Wechsler LR, et al. Teleneurology applications: report of the telemedicine work group of the American academy of neurology. Neurology 2013;80(7):670—6.

[73] Switzer JA, et al. A telestroke network enhances recruitment into acute stroke clinical trials. Stroke 2010;41(3):566—9.

[74] Bunnell BE, et al. An exploration of useful telemedicine-based resources for clinical research. Telemed J E Health 2020;26(1):51—65.

[75] Fonarow GC, et al. Door-to-needle times for tissue plasminogen activator administration and clinical outcomes in acute ischemic stroke before and after a quality improvement initiative. JAMA 2014;311(16):1632—40.

[76] Fonarow GC, et al. Characteristics, performance measures, and in-hospital outcomes of the first one million stroke and transient ischemic attack admissions in get with the guidelines-stroke. Circ Cardiovasc Qual Outcomes 2010;3(3):291—302.

[77] Chalouhi N, et al. Intravenous tissue plasminogen activator administration in community hospitals facilitated by telestroke service. Neurosurgery 2013;73(4):667—71. Discussion 671-2.

[78] Switzer JA, Levine SR, Hess DC. Telestroke 10 years later—'telestroke 2.0'. Cerebrovasc Dis 2009;28(4):323—30.

[79] Switzer JA, Hess DC. Development of regional programs to speed treatment of stroke. Curr Neurol Neurosci Rep 2008;8(1):35—42.

[80] Switzer JA, et al. A web-based telestroke system facilitates rapid treatment of acute ischemic stroke patients in rural emergency departments. J Emerg Med 2009;36(1):12—8.

[81] Meyer BC, et al. Assessment of long-term outcomes for the STRokE DOC telemedicine trial. J Stroke Cerebrovasc Dis 2012;21(4):259—64.

[82] Meyer BC, Demaerschalk BM. Telestroke network fundamentals. J Stroke Cerebrovasc Dis 2012;21(7):521—9.

[83] Meyer BC. Telestroke evolution: from maximization to optimization. Stroke 2012;43(8):2029—30.

[84] Audebert H. Telestroke: effective networking. Lancet Neurol 2006;5(3):279—82.

[85] Audebert HJ, et al. Is mobile teleconsulting equivalent to hospital-based telestroke services? Stroke 2008;39(12):3427—30.

[86] Audebert HJ, et al. Comparison of tissue plasminogen activator administration management between telestroke network hospitals and academic stroke centers: the telemedical pilot project for integrative stroke care in Bavaria/Germany. Stroke 2006;37(7):1822—7.

[87] Audebert HJ, Moulin T. Telestroke: the use of telemedicine in stroke care. Preface. Cerebrovasc Dis 2009;27(Suppl 4):V—VI.

[88] Audebert HJ, Schwamm L. Telestroke: scientific results. Cerebrovasc Dis 2009;27(Suppl 4):15—20.

[89] Sairanen T, et al. Two years of finnish telestroke: thrombolysis at spokes equal to that at the hub. Neurology 2011;76(13):1145—52.

[90] Zaidi SF, et al. Telestroke-guided intravenous tissue-type plasminogen activator treatment achieves a similar clinical outcome as thrombolysis at a comprehensive stroke center. Stroke 2011;42(11):3291–3.

[91] Saadi A, Mateen FJ. International issues: teleneurology in humanitarian crises: Lessons from the Medecins Sans Frontieres experience. Neurology 2017;89(3):e16–9.

[92] Dorsey ER, et al. Teleneurology and mobile technologies: the future of neurological care. Nat Rev Neurol 2018;14(5):285–97.

[93] Howard IM, Kaufman MS. Telehealth applications for outpatients with neuromuscular or musculoskeletal disorders. Muscle Nerve 2018;58(4):475–85.

[94] Association AT. ATA's quick-start guide to telehealth during a health crisis. 2020.

[95] Patel UK, et al. Multidisciplinary approach and outcomes of tele-neurology: a review. Cureus 2019;11(4):e4410.

[96] Smith WR, et al. Implementation guide for rapid integration of an outpatient telemedicine program during the COVID-19 pandemic. J Am Coll Surg 2020;231(2):216–222 e2.

[97] Elson MJ, et al. Telemedicine for Parkinson's disease: limited engagement between local clinicians and remote specialists. Telemed J E Health 2018;24(9):722–4.

[98] O'Carroll CB, et al. Robotic telepresence versus standardly supervised stroke alert team assessments. Telemed J E Health 2015;21(3):151–6.

[99] Velasquez SE, Chaves-Carballo E, Nelson EL. Pediatric teleneurology: a model of epilepsy care for rural populations. Pediatr Neurol 2016;64:32–7.

[100] Lo MD, Gospe Jr SM. Telemedicine and child neurology. J Child Neurol 2019;34(1):22–6.

[101] Kvedar J, Coye MJ, Everett W. Connected health: a review of technologies and strategies to improve patient care with telemedicine and telehealth. Health Aff (Millwood) 2014;33(2):194–9.

[102] health IT, 2020. Available from: https://www.healthit.gov/faq/what-are-technical-infrastructure-requirements-telehealth.

[103] Telemedicine technology. 2020. Available from: https://www.aaaai.org/practice-resources/running-your-practice/practice-management-resources/Telemedicine/technology#:~:text=1.,Mbps%20(Megabits%2Fsec).

[104] Audebert HJ, et al. Telemedicine for safe and extended use of thrombolysis in stroke: the telemedic pilot project for integrative stroke care (TEMPiS) in Bavaria. Stroke 2005;36(2):287–91.

[105] Demaerschalk BM, et al. Efficacy of telemedicine for stroke: pooled analysis of the stroke team remote evaluation using a digital observation camera (STRokE DOC) and STRokE DOC Arizona telestroke trials. Telemed J E Health 2012;18(3):230–7.

[106] Uscher-Pines L, et al. What drives greater assimilation of telestroke in emergency departments? J Stroke Cerebrovasc Dis 2020;29(12):105310.

[107] Demaerschalk BM, et al. American telemedicine association: telestroke guidelines. Telemed J E Health 2017;23(5):376–89.

[108] Donabedian A. The quality of medical care. Science 1978;200(4344):856–64.

[109] McIntyre D, Rogers L, Heier EJ. Overview, history, and objectives of performance measurement. Health Care Financ Rev 2001;22(3):7–21.

[110] Donabedian A. The role of outcomes in quality assessment and assurance. QRB Qual Rev Bull 1992;18(11):356–60.

[111] Demaerschalk BM. Telestrokologists: treating stroke patients here, there, and everywhere with telemedicine. Semin Neurol 2010;30(5):477–91.

[112] Demaerschalk BM. Seamless integrated stroke telemedicine systems of care: a potential solution for acute stroke care delivery delays and inefficiencies. Stroke 2011;42(6):1507–8.

[113] Demaerschalk BM. Telemedicine or telephone consultation in patients with acute stroke. Curr Neurol Neurosci Rep 2011;11(1):42—51.

[114] Sheth KN, et al. Drip and ship thrombolytic therapy for acute ischemic stroke: use, temporal trends, and outcomes. Stroke 2015;46(3):732—9.

[115] Langhorne P, et al. Stroke systems of care in high-income countries: what is optimal? Lancet 2020;396(10260):1433—42.

[116] Meyer D, et al. A stroke care model at an academic, comprehensive stroke center during the 2020 COVID-19 pandemic. J Stroke Cerebrovasc Dis 2020;29(8):104927.

[117] Klein KE, et al. Teleneurocritical care and telestroke. Crit Care Clin 2015;31(2):197—224.

[118] Barrett KM, Freeman WD. Emerging subspecialties in neurology: neurohospitalist. Neurology 2010;74(2):e9—10.

[119] Freeman WD, Josephson SA. The birth of neurohospitalists. Neurohospitalist 2011;1(1):5—7.

[120] Lyden PD. Stroke, research and science in the time of COVID. Stroke 2020;51(9):2613—4.

[121] Office of civil rights HHS COVID-19 pandemic. 2020. Available from: https://www.hhs.gov/about/news/2020/03/17/ocr-announces-notification-of-enforcement-discretion-for-telehealth-remote-communications-during-the-covid-19.html.

[122] Zhao J, et al. Impact of the COVID-19 epidemic on stroke care and potential solutions. Stroke 2020;51(7):1996—2001.

[123] Zhao J, Rudd A, Liu R. Challenges and potential solutions of stroke care during the Coronavirus disease 2019 (COVID-19) outbreak. Stroke 2020;51(5):1356—7.

[124] Center for public health policy. 2020. Available from: https://www.cchpca.org/.

[125] 2020. Available from: https://www.imlcc.org/information-for-physicians/.

[126] Koonin LM, et al. Trends in the use of telehealth during the emergence of the COVID-19 pandemic - United States, January—March 2020. MMWR Morb Mortal Wkly Rep 2020;69(43):1595—9.

[127] van Doremalen N, et al. Aerosol and surface stability of HCoV-19 (SARS-CoV-2) compared to SARS-CoV-1. medRxiv 2020.

[128] van Doremalen N, et al. Aerosol and surface stability of SARS-CoV-2 as compared with SARS-CoV-1. N Engl J Med 2020;382(16):1564—7.

[129] Nguyen TN, et al. Mechanical thrombectomy in the era of the COVID-19 pandemic: emergency preparedness for neuroscience teams: a guidance statement from the society of vascular and interventional neurology. Stroke 2020;51(6):1896—901.

[130] Smith MS, et al. Endovascular therapy for patients with acute ischemic stroke during the COVID-19 pandemic: a proposed algorithm. Stroke 2020;51(6):1902—9.

[131] Huang JF, et al. Telestroke in the time of COVID-19: the Mayo clinic experience. Mayo Clin Proc 2020;95(8):1704—8.

[132] Jasne AS, et al. Stroke code presentations, interventions, and outcomes before and during the COVID-19 pandemic. Stroke 2020;51(9):2664—73.

[133] Shah SO, et al. Rapid decline in telestroke consults in the setting of COVID-19. Telemed J E Health 2021;27(2):227—30.

[134] Nesbitt TS, et al. Telehealth at UC Davis–a 20-year experience. Telemed J E Health 2013;19(5):357—62.

[135] Utidjian L, Abramson E. Pediatric telehealth: opportunities and challenges. Pediatr Clin North Am 2016;63(2):367—78.

[136] Reimbursement. The Robert J. Waters center for telehealth and e-health law. September 24, 2020. Available from: http://ctel.org/expertise/reimbursement.

[137] George BP, et al. Telemedicine in leading US neurology departments. Neurohospitalist 2012;2(4):123—8.

[138] Higgins CA, Conrath DW, Dunn EV. Provider acceptance of telemedicine systems in remote areas of Ontario. J Fam Pract 1984;18(2):285—9.

[139] Uscher-Pines L, Kahn JM. Barriers and facilitators to pediatric emergency telemedicine in the United States. Telemed J E Health 2014;20(11):990—6.

[140] Rogove H, Stetina K. Practice challenges of intensive care unit telemedicine. Crit Care Clin 2015;31(2):319—34.

[141] Rogove HJ, et al. Barriers to telemedicine: survey of current users in acute care units. Telemed J E Health 2012;18(1):48—53.

[142] Cranen K, et al. Toward patient-centered telerehabilitation design: understanding chronic pain patients' preferences for web-based exercise telerehabilitation using a discrete choice experiment. J Med Internet Res 2017;19(1):e26.

[143] Cranen K, et al. Change of patients' perceptions of telemedicine after brief use. Telemed J E Health 2011;17(7):530—5.

[144] Conn DK, et al. Program evaluation of a telepsychiatry service for older adults connecting a university-affiliated geriatric center to a rural psychogeriatric outreach service in Northwest Ontario, Canada. Int Psychogeriatr 2013;25(11):1795—800.

[145] Lam K, et al. Assessing telemedicine unreadiness among older adults in the United States during the COVID-19 pandemic. JAMA Intern Med 2020.

[146] Cimperman M, et al. Older adults' perceptions of home telehealth services. Telemed J E Health 2013;19(10):786—90.

[147] Cimperman M, Makovec Brencic M, Trkman P. Analyzing older users' home telehealth services acceptance behavior-applying an extended UTAUT model. Int J Med Inform 2016;90:22—31.

[148] Donaghy E, et al. Acceptability, benefits, and challenges of video consulting: a qualitative study in primary care. Br J Gen Pract 2019;69(686):e586—94.

[149] Agarwal S, Warburton EA. Teleneurology: is it really at a distance? J Neurol 2011;258(6):971—81.

[150] Katz HP, et al. Patient safety and telephone medicine: some lessons from closed claim case review. J Gen Intern Med 2008;23(5):517—22.

[151] Freeman WD, et al. Future neurohospitalist: teleneurohospitalist. Neurohospitalist 2012;2(4):132—43.

[152] R C. Informed refusal the Doctor's company. 2020.

[153] Marcin JP, et al. Using telemedicine to provide pediatric subspecialty care to children with special health care needs in an underserved rural community. Pediatrics 2004;113(1 Pt 1):1—6.

[154] Fanale CV, Demaerschalk BM. Telestroke network business model strategies. J Stroke Cerebrovasc Dis 2012;21(7):530—4.

[155] Mistry H. Systematic review of studies of the cost-effectiveness of telemedicine and telecare. Changes in the economic evidence over twenty years. J Telemed Telecare 2012;18(1):1—6.

[156] Medicare benefits policy manual, publication 100—02, Chapter 15. 2013. Available from: Center for Medicare and Medicaid Services Web site, http://www.cms.gov/Regulations-and-Guidance/Guidance/Manuals/downloads/bp102c15.pdf.

[157] Aita MC, et al. Obstacles and solutions in the implementation of telestroke: billing, licensing, and legislation. Stroke 2013;44(12):3602—6.

[158] Silva GS, et al. The status of telestroke in the United States: a survey of currently active stroke telemedicine programs. Stroke 2012;43(8):2078—85.

[159] Demaerschalk BM, et al. Smartphone teleradiology application is successfully incorporated into a telestroke network environment. Stroke 2012;43(11):3098—101.

[160] Macedo FS, et al. Evaluation of usability, perception of usefulness, and efficiency of an application in interpreting imaging examinations and supporting decision-making in orthopedics. Telemed J E Health 2020.

[161] Rachel Patrizzo. Cybersecurity insurance for medical practice-the basics. The Doctor's Company; 2020.

[162] Saver JL. Time is brain–quantified. Stroke 2006;37(1):263–6.

[163] Acker 3rd JE, et al. Implementation strategies for emergency medical services within stroke systems of care: a policy statement from the American Heart Association/American Stroke Association Expert Panel on Emergency Medical Services Systems and the Stroke Council. Stroke 2007;38(11):3097–115.

[164] Audebert HJ, et al. Effects of the implementation of a telemedical stroke network: the telemedic pilot project for integrative stroke care (TEMPiS) in Bavaria, Germany. Lancet Neurol 2006;5(9):742–8.

[165] Hov MR, et al. Interpretation of brain CT scans in the field by critical care physicians in a mobile stroke unit. J Neuroimaging 2018;28(1):106–11.

[166] Audebert H, et al. The PRE-hospital stroke treatment organization. Int J Stroke 2017;12(9):932–40.

[167] Ebinger M, et al. Prehospital thrombolysis: a manual from Berlin. J Vis Exp 2013;(81):e50534.

[168] Ebinger M, et al. PHANTOM-S: the prehospital acute neurological therapy and optimization of medical care in stroke patients - study. Int J Stroke 2012;7(4):348–53.

[169] Moodie M, et al. Economic evaluation of Australian stroke services: a prospective, multicenter study comparing dedicated stroke units with other care modalities. Stroke 2006;37(11):2790–5.

[170] Weber JE, et al. Prehospital thrombolysis in acute stroke: results of the PHANTOM-S pilot study. Neurology 2013;80(2):163–8.

[171] Dietrich M, et al. Is prehospital treatment of acute stroke too expensive? An economic evaluation based on the first trial. Cerebrovasc Dis 2014;38(6):457–63.

[172] Wu TC, et al. Telemedicine can replace the neurologist on a mobile stroke unit. Stroke 2017;48(2):493–6.

[173] Harris J. A review of mobile stroke units. J Neurol 2020.

[174] Itrat A, et al. Telemedicine in prehospital stroke evaluation and thrombolysis: taking stroke treatment to the doorstep. JAMA Neurol 2016;73(2):162–8.

[175] Fassbender K, et al. Mobile stroke units for prehospital thrombolysis, triage, and beyond: benefits and challenges. Lancet Neurol 2017;16(3):227–37.

[176] Goyal M, Demchuk AM, Hill MD. Endovascular therapy for ischemic stroke. N Engl J Med 2015;372(24):2366.

[177] Campbell BC, et al. Endovascular therapy proven for stroke - finally! Heart Lung Circ 2015;24(8):733–5.

[178] Berkhemer OA, et al. Endovascular therapy for ischemic stroke. N Engl J Med 2015;372(24):2363.

[179] Adeoye O, et al. Geographic access to acute stroke care in the United States. Stroke 2014;45(10):3019–24.

[180] Adeoye O, et al. Recommendations for the establishment of stroke systems of care: a 2019 update. Stroke 2019;50(7):e187–210.

[181] Prabhakaran S, et al. Transfer delay is a major factor limiting the use of intra-arterial treatment in acute ischemic stroke. Stroke 2011;42(6):1626–30.

[182] Pedragosa A, et al. Impact of telemedicine on acute management of stroke patients undergoing endovascular procedures. Cerebrovasc Dis 2012;34(5-6):436–42.

[183] Barlinn J, et al. Acute endovascular treatment delivery to ischemic stroke patients transferred within a telestroke network: a retrospective observational study. Int J Stroke 2017;12(5):502–9.

[184] Boulos MN, et al. Mobile medical and health apps: state of the art, concerns, regulatory control and certification. Online J Public Health Inform 2014;5(3):229.

[185] Nogueira RG, et al. The FAST-ED app: a smartphone platform for the field triage of patients with stroke. Stroke 2017;48(5):1278—84.

[186] Calleja-Castillo JM, Gonzalez-Calderon G. WhatsApp in stroke systems: current use and regulatory concerns. Front Neurol 2018;9:388.

[187] Wilson JL, Eriksson CO, Williams CN. Endovascular therapy in pediatric stroke: utilization, patient characteristics, and outcomes. Pediatr Neurol 2017;69:87—92 e2.

[188] Yaeger KA, et al. Emerging technologies in optimizing pre-intervention workflow for acute stroke. Neurosurgery 2019;85(suppl 1):S9—17.

[189] Takao H, et al. Primary salvage survey of the interference of radiowaves emitted by smartphones on medical equipment. Health Phys 2016;111(4):381—92.

[190] Kageji T, et al. Drip-and-ship thrombolytic therapy supported by the telestroke system for acute ischemic stroke patients living in medically under-served areas. Neurol Med Chir (Tokyo) 2016;56(12):753—8.

[191] Mokin M, et al. Recent endovascular stroke trials and their impact on stroke systems of care. J Am Coll Cardiol 2016;67(22):2645—55.

[192] Silva JNA, et al. Emerging applications of virtual reality in cardiovascular medicine. JACC Basic Transl Sci 2018;3(3):420—30.

[193] Hilty DM, et al. Virtual reality, telemedicine, web and data processing innovations in medical and psychiatric education and clinical care. Acad Psychiatry 2006;30(6):528—33.

[194] Garcia-Bravo S, et al. Virtual reality and video games in cardiac rehabilitation programs. A systematic review. Disabil Rehabil 2019:1—10.

[195] Eckert M, Volmerg JS, Friedrich CM. Augmented reality in medicine: systematic and bibliographic review. JMIR Mhealth Uhealth 2019;7(4):e10967.

[196] Mazzaccaro D, Nano G. The use of virtual reality for carotid artery stenting (CAS) training in type I and type III aortic arches. Ann Ital Chir 2012;83(2):81—5.

[197] Willaert WI, et al. Role of patient-specific virtual reality rehearsal in carotid artery stenting. Br J Surg 2012;99(9):1304—13.

[198] Davids J, et al. Simulation for skills training in neurosurgery: a systematic review, meta-analysis, and analysis of progressive scholarly acceptance. Neurosurg Rev 2020.

[199] Johnson T, et al. Virtual reality use for symptom management in palliative care: a pilot study to assess user perceptions. J Palliat Med 2020;23(9):1233—8.

[200] Coupar F, et al. Home-based therapy programmes for upper limb functional recovery following stroke. Cochrane Database Syst Rev 2012;(5):CD006755.

[201] Coupar F, et al. Simultaneous bilateral training for improving arm function after stroke. Cochrane Database Syst Rev 2010;(4):CD006432.

[202] Langhorne P, Coupar F, Pollock A. Motor recovery after stroke: a systematic review. Lancet Neurol 2009;8(8):741—54.

[203] Espay AJ, et al. At-home training with closed-loop augmented-reality cueing device for improving gait in patients with Parkinson disease. J Rehabil Res Dev 2010;47(6):573—81.

[204] Henderson A, Korner-Bitensky N, Levin M. Virtual reality in stroke rehabilitation: a systematic review of its effectiveness for upper limb motor recovery. Top Stroke Rehabil 2007;14(2):52—61.

[205] Henderson S, Feiner S. Opportunistic tangible user interfaces for augmented reality. IEEE Trans Vis Comput Graph 2010;16(1):4—16.

[206] Saposnik G, et al. Efficacy and safety of non-immersive virtual reality exercising in stroke rehabilitation (EVREST): a randomised, multicentre, single-blind, controlled trial. Lancet Neurol 2016;15(10):1019—27.

[207] Saposnik G, Levin M, Outcome Research Canada Working G. Virtual reality in stroke rehabilitation: a meta-analysis and implications for clinicians. Stroke 2011;42(5):1380—6.

[208] Saposnik G, et al. Effectiveness of virtual reality exercises in stroke rehabilitation (EVREST): rationale, design, and protocol of a pilot randomized clinical trial assessing the Wii gaming system. Int J Stroke 2010;5(1):47—51.

[209] Saposnik G, et al. Effectiveness of virtual reality using Wii gaming technology in stroke rehabilitation: a pilot randomized clinical trial and proof of principle. Stroke 2010;41(7):1477—84.

[210] Piron L, et al. Exercises for paretic upper limb after stroke: a combined virtual-reality and telemedicine approach. J Rehabil Med 2009;41(12):1016—102.

[211] Johansson T, Wild C. Telerehabilitation in stroke care–a systematic review. J Telemed Telecare 2011;17(1):1—6.

[212] Kellner CP, et al. The VITAL study and overall pooled analysis with the VIPS non-invasive stroke detection device. J Neurointerv Surg 2018;10(11):1079—84.

[213] Jiang F, et al. Artificial intelligence in healthcare: past, present and future. Stroke Vasc Neurol 2017;2(4):230—43.

[214] Hassan AE, et al. Early experience utilizing artificial intelligence shows significant reduction in transfer times and length of stay in a hub and spoke model. Interv Neuroradiol 2020;26(5):615—22.

[215] Hassan AE. New technology add-on payment (NTAP) for Viz LVO: a win for stroke care. J Neurointerv Surg 2020.

[216] Panesar SS, et al. Telerobotic stroke intervention: a novel solution to the care dissemination dilemma. J Neurosurg 2019;132(3):971—8.

[217] Britz GW, et al. Neuroendovascular-specific engineering modifications to the Cor-Path GRX Robotic System. J Neurosurg 2019:1—7.

[218] Desai VR, et al. Initial experience in a pig model of robotic-assisted intracranial arteriovenous malformation (AVM) embolization. Oper Neurosurg (Hagerstown) 2020;19(2):205—9.

[219] Mahmud E, et al. Demonstration of the safety and feasibility of robotically assisted percutaneous coronary intervention in complex coronary lesions: results of the CORA-PCI study (complex robotically assisted percutaneous coronary intervention). JACC Cardiovasc Interv 2017;10(13):1320—7.

[220] Wegermann ZK, Swaminathan RV, Rao SV. Cath lab robotics: paradigm change in interventional cardiology? Curr Cardiol Rep 2019;21(10):119.

[221] Jabbour P, et al. Stroke in the robotic era. World Neurosurg 2010;73(6):603—4.

[222] Dobkin BH. Wearable motion sensors to continuously measure real-world physical activities. Curr Opin Neurol 2013;26(6):602—8.

[223] Dobkin BH, Martinez C. Wearable sensors to monitor, enable feedback, and measure outcomes of activity and practice. Curr Neurol Neurosci Rep 2018;18(12):87.

[224] Siwicki B. A guide to connected health device and remote patient monitoring vendors. HIMSS [ehealth] 2020. Available from: https://www.healthcareitnews.com/news/guide-connected-health-device-and-remote-patient-monitoring-vendors.

[225] Kvedar JC. Evidence for the effectiveness of digital health. NPJ Digit Med 2020;3:34.

[226] Kvedar JC, Fogel AL. mHealth advances clinical research, bit by bit. Nat Biotechnol 2017;35(4):337—9.

[227] Reed MJ, et al. Multi-centre randomised controlled trial of a smart phone-based event recorder alongside standard care versus standard care for patients presenting to the Emergency Department with palpitations and pre-syncope - the IPED (investigation of palpitations in the ED) study: study protocol for a randomised controlled trial. Trials 2018;19(1):711.

[228] Koshy AN, et al. Smart watches for heart rate assessment in atrial arrhythmias. Int J Cardiol 2018;266:124—7.

[229] Saxon LA, et al. Long-term outcome after ICD and CRT implantation and influence of remote device follow-up: the ALTITUDE survival study. Circulation 2010;122(23):2359−67.

[230] Ong MK, et al. Effectiveness of remote patient monitoring after discharge of hospitalized patients with heart failure: the better effectiveness after transition − heart failure (BEAT-HF) randomized clinical trial. JAMA Intern Med 2016;176(3):310−8.

[231] Ono M, Varma N. Remote monitoring to improve long-term prognosis in heart failure patients with implantable cardioverter-defibrillators. Expert Rev Med Devices 2017;14(5):335−42.

[232] Ono M, Varma N. Remote monitoring for chronic disease management: atrial fibrillation and heart failure. Card Electrophysiol Clin 2018;10(1):43−58.

[233] Varma N, et al. Automatic remote monitoring utilizing daily transmissions: transmission reliability and implantable cardioverter defibrillator battery longevity in the TRUST trial. Europace 2018;20(4):622−8.

[234] Varma N, et al. HRS/EHRA/APHRS/LAHRS/ACC/AHA worldwide practice update for telehealth and arrhythmia monitoring during and after a pandemic. J Arrhythm 2020.

[235] Behar J, et al. Remote health diagnosis and monitoring in the time of COVID-19. Physiol Meas 2020.

[236] Goldberg L, et al. Usability and accessibility in consumer health informatics current trends and future challenges. Am J Prev Med 2011;40(5 Suppl 2):S187−97.

[237] El-Gayar O, et al. Mobile applications for diabetes self-management: status and potential. J Diabetes Sci Technol 2013;7(1):247−62.

[238] Cabitza F. Introducing a composite index of information quality for medical web sites. Stud Health Technol Inform 2012;180:1162−4.

[239] Noorian AR, et al. Use of wearable technology in remote evaluation of acute stroke patients: feasibility and reliability of a google glass-based device. J Stroke Cerebrovasc Dis 2019;28(10):104258.

[240] Munusamy T, et al. Telemedicine via smart glasses in critical care of the neurosurgical patient - a COVID-19 pandemic preparedness and response in neurosurgery. World Neurosurg 2020.

[241] Ye J, et al. A telemedicine wound care model using 4G with smart phones or smart glasses: a pilot study. Medicine (Baltimore) 2016;95(31):e4198.

[242] Roberts DJ, et al. Estimating the gaze of a virtuality human. IEEE Trans Vis Comput Graph 2013;19(4):681−90.

[243] Lim JH, et al. Cholecystectomy using the Revo-i robotic surgical system from Korea: the first clinical study. Updates Surg 2020.

[244] Agarwal DK, et al. Initial experience with da Vinci single-port robot-assisted radical prostatectomies. Eur Urol 2020;77(3):373−9.

[245] Fiacchini G, et al. Is the Da Vinci Xi system a real improvement for oncologic transoral robotic surgery? A systematic review of the literature. J Robot Surg 2020.

[246] Moyle W, et al. Potential of telepresence robots to enhance social connectedness in older adults with dementia: an integrative review of feasibility. Int Psychogeriatr 2017;29(12):1951−64.

[247] Moyle W, et al. Care staff perceptions of a social robot called Paro and a look-alike Plush Toy: a descriptive qualitative approach. Aging Ment Health 2018;22(3):330−5.

[248] Moyle W, et al. "She had a smile on her face as wide as the great Australian bite": a qualitative examination of family perceptions of a therapeutic robot and a plush toy. Gerontologist 2019;59(1):177−85.

[249] Moyle W, et al. Connecting the person with dementia and family: a feasibility study of a telepresence robot. BMC Geriatr 2014;14:7.

[250] Moyle W, et al. Using a therapeutic companion robot for dementia symptoms in long-term care: reflections from a cluster-RCT. Aging Ment Health 2019;23(3):329—36.

[251] Al-Khathaami AM, et al. Cultural acceptance of robotic telestroke medicine among patients and healthcare providers in Saudi Arabia. Results of a pilot study. Neuro-sciences (Riyadh) 2015;20(1):27—30.

[252] Yang JP, et al. Targeting telestroke: benchmarking time performance in telestroke consultations. J Stroke Cerebrovasc Dis 2013;22(4):470—5.

[253] Lai F. Stroke networks based on robotic telepresence. J Telemed Telecare 2009;15(3):135—6.

[254] Vespa P. Robotic telepresence in the intensive care unit. Crit Care 2005;9(4):319—20.

[255] Vespa PM. Multimodality monitoring and telemonitoring in neurocritical care: from microdialysis to robotic telepresence. Curr Opin Crit Care 2005;11(2):133—8.

[256] Vespa PM, et al. Intensive care unit robotic telepresence facilitates rapid physician response to unstable patients and decreased cost in neurointensive care. Surg Neurol 2007;67(4):331—7.

[257] Patel TM, Shah SC, Pancholy SB. Long distance tele-robotic-assisted percutaneous coronary intervention: a report of first-in-human experience. EClinicalMedicine 2019;14:53—8.

[258] Wier LM, et al. Overview of children in the emergency department, 2010: statistical brief #157, in healthcare cost and utilization project (HCUP) statistical briefs. 2006. Rockville (MD).

[259] McDermott KW, Stocks C, Freeman WJ. Overview of pediatric emergency department visits, 2015: statistical brief #242, in healthcare cost and utilization project (HCUP) statistical briefs. 2006. Rockville (MD).

[260] Berger E. Growing pains: report notes pediatric emergencies need greater emphasis. Ann Emerg Med 2006;48(2):143—4.

[261] Dharmar M, et al. Telemedicine consultations and medication errors in rural emergency departments. Pediatrics 2013;132(6):1090—7.

[262] Dharmar M, et al. Impact of critical care telemedicine consultations on children in rural emergency departments. Crit Care Med 2013;41(10):2388—95.

[263] Dharmar M, et al. The financial impact of a pediatric telemedicine program: a children's hospital's perspective. Telemed J E Health 2013;19(7):502—8.

[264] Brova M, et al. Pediatric telemedicine use in United States emergency departments. Acad Emerg Med 2018;25(12):1427—32.

[265] The role of telehealth in an evolving health care environment: workshop summary. 2012. Washington (DC).

[266] Committee On Pediatric W, et al. The use of telemedicine to address access and physician workforce shortages. Pediatrics 2015;136(1):202—9.

[267] Heath B, et al. Pediatric critical care telemedicine in rural underserved emergency departments. Pediatr Crit Care Med 2009;10(5):588—91.

[268] Marcin JP, et al. Changes in diagnosis, treatment, and clinical improvement among patients receiving telemedicine consultations. Telemed J E Health 2005;11(1):36—43.

[269] Marcin JP, et al. Use of telemedicine to provide pediatric critical care inpatient consultations to underserved rural Northern California. J Pediatr 2004;144(3):375—80.

[270] Finley JP, Warren AE. Recent article by Mahnke et al describing pediatric murmur assessment using remote digital recordings of heart sounds. Clin Pediatr (Phila) 2009;48(7):789.

[271] Garingo A, et al. "Tele-rounding" with a remotely controlled mobile robot in the neonatal intensive care unit. J Telemed Telecare 2016;22(2):132—8.

[272] Garingo A, et al. The use of mobile robotic telemedicine technology in the neonatal intensive care unit. J Perinatol 2012;32(1):55—63.

[273] Guzman CS, Pignatiello A. The benefits of implementing telepsychiatry in the Brazilian mental health system. Braz J Psychiatry 2008;30(3):300—1.

[274] Hilgart JS, et al. Telegenetics: a systematic review of telemedicine in genetics services. Genet Med 2012;14(9):765—76.

[275] Pignatiello A, et al. Child and youth telepsychiatry in rural and remote primary care. Child Adolesc Psychiatr Clin N Am 2011;20(1):13—28.

[276] Satou GM, et al. Telemedicine in pediatric cardiology: a scientific statement from the American Heart Association. Circulation 2017;135(11):e648—78.

[277] Shivji S, et al. Pediatric surgery telehealth: patient and clinician satisfaction. Pediatr Surg Int 2011;27(5):523—6.

[278] Rametta SC, et al. Analyzing 2,589 child neurology telehealth encounters necessitated by the COVID-19 pandemic. Neurology 2020;95(9):e1257—66.

[279] Ray KN, et al. Telemedicine and outpatient subspecialty visits among pediatric medicaid beneficiaries. Acad Pediatr 2020;20(5):642—51.

[280] Weber DJ, et al. Training in neurology: rapid implementation of cross-institutional neurology resident education in the time of COVID-19. Neurology 2020.

[281] McConnochie KM. Potential of telemedicine in pediatric primary care. Pediatr Rev 2006;27(9):e58—65.

[282] McConnochie KM. Pursuit of value in connected healthcare. Telemed J E Health 2015;21(11):863—9.

[283] McConnochie KM, et al. Effectiveness and safety of acute care telemedicine for children with regular and special healthcare needs. Telemed J E Health 2015;21(8):611—21.

[284] McConnochie KM, et al. Care offered by an information-rich pediatric acute illness connected care model. Telemed J E Health 2016;22(6):465—72.

[285] McConnochie KM, et al. Telemedicine reduces absence resulting from illness in urban child care: evaluation of an innovation. Pediatrics 2005;115(5):1273—82.

[286] Mallick AA, et al. Childhood arterial ischaemic stroke incidence, presenting features, and risk factors: a prospective population-based study. Lancet Neurol 2014;13(1):35—43.

[287] Lehman LL, et al. What will improve pediatric acute stroke care? Stroke 2019;50(2):249—56.

[288] Agrawal N, et al. Imaging data reveal a higher pediatric stroke incidence than prior US estimates. Stroke 2009;40(11):3415—21.

[289] Fullerton HJ, et al. Risk of stroke in children: ethnic and gender disparities. Neurology 2003;61(2):189—94.

[290] Berkhemer OA, Majoie CB, Dippel DW. Intraarterial treatment for acute ischemic stroke. N Engl J Med 2015;372(12):1178—9.

[291] Bernard TJ, et al. Preparing for a "pediatric stroke alert". Pediatr Neurol 2016;56:18—24.

[292] Bernard TJ, et al. Emergence of the primary pediatric stroke center: impact of the thrombolysis in pediatric stroke trial. Stroke 2014;45(7):2018—23.

[293] Bhatia K, et al. Mechanical thrombectomy in pediatric stroke: systematic review, individual patient data meta-analysis, and case series. J Neurosurg Pediatr 2019:1—14.

[294] Ray KN, et al. Clinician attitudes toward adoption of pediatric emergency telemedicine in rural hospitals. Pediatr Emerg Care 2017;33(4):250—7.

[295] Yager PH, et al. Nighttime telecommunication between remote staff intensivists and bedside personnel in a pediatric intensive care unit: a retrospective study. Crit Care Med 2012;40(9):2700—3.

[296] Mackay MT, et al. Differentiating childhood stroke from mimics in the emergency department. Stroke 2016;47(10):2476—81.

[297] Gabis LV, Yangala R, Lenn NJ. Time lag to diagnosis of stroke in children. Pediatrics 2002;110(5):924—8.

[298] Srinivasan J, et al. Delayed recognition of initial stroke in children: need for increased awareness. Pediatrics 2009;124(2):e227—34.

[299] Rafay MF, et al. Delay to diagnosis in acute pediatric arterial ischemic stroke. Stroke 2009;40(1):58—64.

[300] McGlennan C, Ganesan V. Delays in investigation and management of acute arterial ischaemic stroke in children. Dev Med Child Neurol 2008;50(7):537—40.

[301] Mackay MT, et al. Parental care-seeking behavior and prehospital timelines of care in childhood arterial ischemic stroke. Stroke 2016;47(10):2638—40.

[302] Kidwell CS, et al. Identifying stroke in the field. Prospective validation of the Los Angeles prehospital stroke screen (LAPSS). Stroke 2000;31(1):71—6.

[303] Mackay MT, et al. Performance of bedside stroke recognition tools in discriminating childhood stroke from mimics. Neurology 2016;86(23):2154—61.

[304] Neville K, Lo W. Sensitivity and specificity of an adult stroke screening tool in childhood ischemic stroke. Pediatr Neurol 2016;58:53—6.

[305] Brott T, et al. Measurements of acute cerebral infarction: a clinical examination scale. Stroke 1989;20(7):864—70.

[306] Ichord RN, et al. Interrater reliability of the Pediatric National Institutes of Health Stroke Scale (PedNIHSS) in a multicenter study. Stroke 2011;42(3):613—7.

[307] Ferriero DM, et al. Management of stroke in neonates and children: a scientific statement from the American Heart Association/American Stroke Association. Stroke 2019;50(3):e51—96.

[308] Rivkin MJ, et al. Thrombolysis in pediatric stroke study. Stroke 2015;46(3):880—5.

[309] Wharton JD, et al. Pediatric acute stroke protocol implementation and utilization over 7 years. J Pediatr 2020;220:214—220 e1.

[310] Ladner TR, et al. Mechanical thrombectomy for acute stroke in childhood: how much does restricted diffusion matter? BMJ Case Rep 2014;2014.

[311] Ladner TR, et al. Mechanical thrombectomy for acute stroke in childhood: how much does restricted diffusion matter? J Neurointerv Surg 2015;7(12):e40.

[312] Ladner TR, et al. Pediatric acute stroke protocol activation in a children's hospital emergency department. Stroke 2015;46(8):2328—31.

[313] Khan IS, et al. Endovascular thrombolysis for pediatric cerebral sinus venous thrombosis with tissue plasminogen activator and abciximab. J Neurosurg Pediatr 2014;13(1):68—71.

[314] Buompadre MC, et al. Thrombectomy for acute stroke in childhood: a case report, literature review, and recommendations. Pediatr Neurol 2017;66:21—7.

[315] Harrar DB, et al. A stroke alert protocol decreases the time to diagnosis of brain attack symptoms in a pediatric emergency department. J Pediatr 2020;216:136—141 e6.

[316] deVeber GA, et al. Epidemiology and outcomes of arterial ischemic stroke in children: the Canadian pediatric ischemic stroke registry. Pediatr Neurol 2017;69:58—70.

[317] Grunt S, et al. Incidence and outcomes of symptomatic neonatal arterial ischemic stroke. Pediatrics 2015;135(5):e1220—8.

[318] Edwards H, et al. Outcomes following childhood arterial ischaemic stroke: a Delphi Consensus on what parents want from future research. Eur J Paediatr Neurol 2015;19(2):181—7.

[319] Steinlin M, et al. The first three years of the Swiss Neuropaediatric Stroke Registry (SNPSR): a population-based study of incidence, symptoms and risk factors. Neuropediatrics 2005;36(2):90—7.

[320] Burke Jr BL, Hall RW, Section On Telehealth C. Telemedicine: pediatric applications. Pediatrics 2015;136(1):e293—308.

[321] Grefe A, Hsieh D, Joshi C, Joshi S, Mintz M, Segal M, Shahid A. Pediatric neurological examination via telemedicine. 2020.

[322] Al Hussona M, et al. The virtual neurologic exam: instructional videos and guidance for the COVID-19 era. Can J Neurol Sci 2020:1—6.

[323] Craig J, et al. A pilot study of telemedicine for new neurological outpatient referrals. J Telemed Telecare 2000;6(4):225—8.

[324] Craig J, et al. Interactive videoconsultation is a feasible method for neurological in-patient assessment. Eur J Neurol 2000;7(6):699—702.

[325] Craig JJ, et al. Neurological examination is possible using telemedicine. J Telemed Telecare 1999;5(3):177—81.

[326] Demchuk AM, et al. Predictors of good outcome after intravenous tPA for acute ischemic stroke. Neurology 2001;57(3):474—80.

[327] Dosaj A, et al. Rapid implementation of telehealth services during the COVID-19 pandemic. Telemed J E Health 2020.

[328] Woodward MA, et al. Telemedicine for ophthalmic consultation services: use of a portable device and layering information for graders. J Telemed Telecare 2017;23(2):365—70.

[329] Richard JV, et al. Assessment of telestroke capacity in US hospitals. JAMA Neurol 2020;77(8):1035—7.

Index

Printed in the United States
by Baker & Taylor Publisher Services